THE FIRST TWO YEARS

A STUDY OF TWENTY-FIVE BABIES

VOLUME I

POSTURAL AND LOCOMOTOR DEVELOPMENT

UNIVERSITY OF MINNESOTA
THE INSTITUTE OF CHILD WELFARE
MONOGRAPH SERIES NO. VI

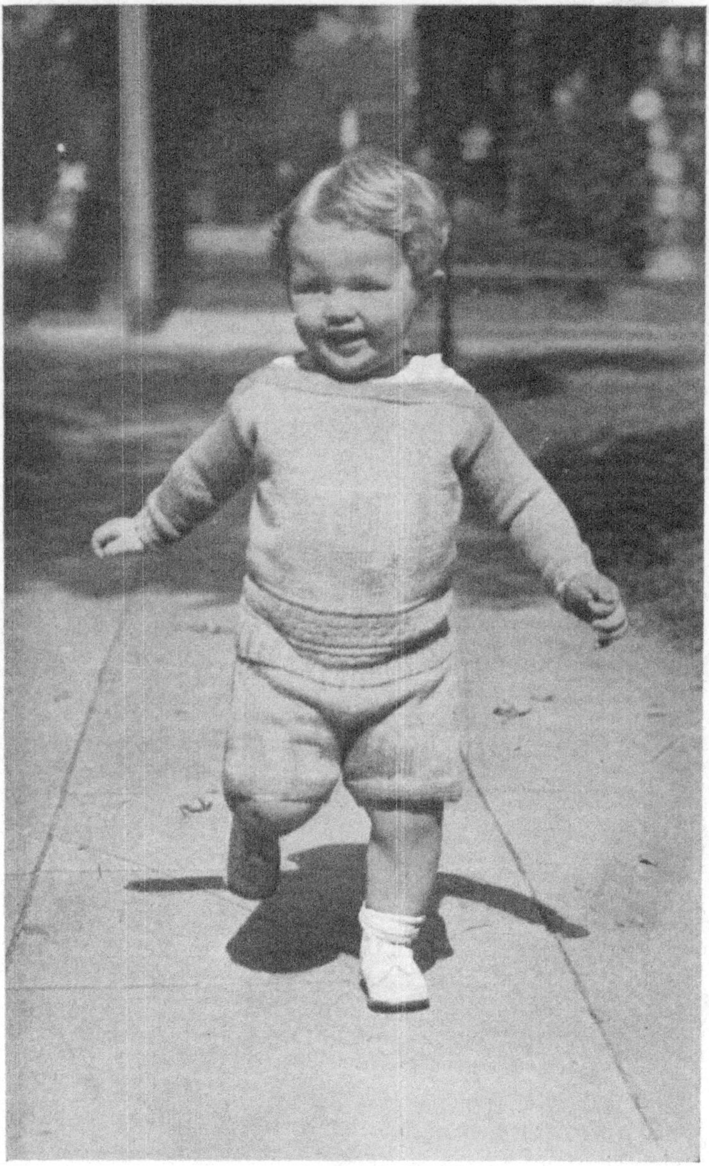

His Morning Constitutional
(Walley at 96 weeks)

THE FIRST TWO YEARS

A STUDY OF TWENTY-FIVE BABIES

By
MARY M. SHIRLEY
Assistant Professor
Institute of Child Welfare
University of Minnesota

VOLUME I

POSTURAL AND LOCOMOTOR DEVELOPMENT

THE UNIVERSITY OF MINNESOTA PRESS
MINNEAPOLIS

PRINTED IN THE UNITED STATES
OF AMERICA

FOREWORD

In the modern approach to the scientific study of the child, observations on the physical and mental development of infants play a prominent part. Within the last five years a number of ambitious investigations have been undertaken and are now finding their way into print. As a result many of the conceptions and points of view previously held are being modified, and much that should contribute to our understanding of the entire course of development is becoming available. Obviously, infant behavior is of particular importance in any genetic view of life.

As the result of a number of investigations in various centers a point of view is evolving that pictures the development of the infant as an orderly process, in which different types of response unfold at successive stages. While the time of the appearance of these various responses varies, the order of events seems to be fairly constant. Furthermore, the appearance of the responses seems to follow a uniform principle, namely that of progress from general and diffuse behavior to specific and organized behavior. At their first appearance responses also seem to have a fluid character — that is, they sometimes appear under appropriate stimulation and sometimes do not — a character that disappears as development proceeds. Where earlier investigators sought fixed and independent units in the early behavior of the infant, students now look upon fixity and specificity of response as terminal rather than initial stages.

In this study Dr. Shirley analyzes the postural and locomotor development of the infant, leaving for two subsequent monographs the study of intellectual development and of personality manifestations. The three monographs will constitute a report on the psychology and behavior of twenty-five infants of whom a study was made by the Institute of Child Welfare over a two-year period. The present monograph is of especial interest because of its analysis of the successive stages of gross motor development as revealed in walking and in major bodily coordinations. For the recording of progress in locomotion an interesting objective technique was developed. The study of the physical growth and physiological development of these infants, which was under the direction of Dr. Edith Boyd, will be presented in a separate monograph.

In undertaking the study the cooperation of twenty-four prospective mothers was obtained. Periodic examinations of the infants were made, first in the hospitals and later in the homes, during a two-year period by a physician, Dr. Boyd, and a psychologist, Dr. Shirley. The mothers kept daily records on prepared forms and supplied much supplementary data. The records obtained through the cooperation of the scientific observers and the mothers give one of the most comprehensive surveys of infant development that has appeared.

On behalf of the Institute of Child Welfare I wish to express our appreciation and gratitude to the mothers who gave such excellent cooperation in the study. Without their active participation it would have been impossible to carry out so long and detailed an investigation. They are pioneers in a type of cooperation between home and laboratory that may contribute much to our knowledge and understanding of children.

John E. Anderson
Director, Institute of Child Welfare
University of Minnesota

ACKNOWLEDGMENTS

To the twenty-four Minneapolis mothers whose babies were the subjects of this study I express my deepest gratitude. Without their gracious cooperation and unflagging interest the study could not have gone forward at all. I wish especially to thank Mrs. Dorothea Lynde Anderson, who read and criticized the manuscript from the mother's point of view.

Dr. Edith Boyd, my coworker in the investigation, has my sincerest appreciation and thanks for her keen observations, her farseeing suggestions, her faithful collaboration, and her friendly criticisms throughout the gathering of the data and the writing of the monograph.

For unstinted financial support of the project and for unlimited freedom in carrying on the research I am under great obligation to the University of Minnesota Institute of Child Welfare and in particular to its director, Dr. John E. Anderson. I am also heavily indebted to Dr. Anderson and to Dr. Florence L. Goodenough for helpful advice during the course of the study and for valuable suggestions and criticisms of the manuscript.

Finally I wish to make grateful acknowledgment to Mrs. Bess Crowder James, Mrs. Helen Gillis Garvey, Miss Ella J. Weig, and Mrs. Dorothy Kenning Wells, who assisted in working up the data, to Mr. Donovan Lawrence, photographer and technician of the institute, and to several graduate students who helped at intervals in the collection and compilation of material.

MARY SHIRLEY

University of Minnesota
June 3, 1930

TABLE OF CONTENTS

LIST OF TABLES

LIST OF FIGURES

LIST OF PLATES

CHAPTER I

NATURE, PURPOSE, AND METHODS OF THE STUDY AS A WHOLE

In the study of childhood the realm of infancy has been least penetrated by the psychologist. Because they have been easily accessible to educators and other investigators, school children have long been studied. With the growth of nursery schools in the last decade preschool children have become increasingly available for systematic observation. But babies have always been stay-at-home bodies, and there they have been so hedged about by parental care that they have seldom come under the scrutiny of science. Not that the scientist considers infants unworthy of his attention. A creature who more than triples his original seven pounds and who progresses from squirming to walking and from futile crying to communicative talking, all in the course of two short years, is certainly well worth study.

The first two years are a period of very rapid physical growth, as well as the period of the beginnings of motor skills and speech. During babyhood traits of personality put in their appearance, and intellectual and emotional trends come to light. Many careful observers hold that in these earliest years habits are formed that follow the individual throughout life. Scientific information on babies is bound to lead to a clearer understanding of children, youths, and adults.

With the aim of filling in some of the gaps in our present knowledge of children under nursery school age the University of Minnesota Institute of Child Welfare early laid plans for a study of infancy. Mindful of the difficulties confronting one who tries to piece together a complete picture of babyhood from the mosaical fragments of data on many different babies gathered by many scientists, members of the Institute formulated two requirements for the study: first, that the same babies be observed repeatedly over a long period of time by the same observers; and second, that the many aspects of development, anatomical, physical, motor, intellectual, and emotional, be studied simultaneously. In seeking a method for the study these two aims were made the primary consideration.

The infant-study project got under way in the summer of 1927. Many plans for obtaining babies for the study were discussed, and at last the method of home visiting was decided upon as the only practical way of keeping in contact with the same children over a two-year period. Many of the difficulties and disadvantages of going into a home to make scientific observations on its youngest member will be readily apparent. Before going on to a fuller description of the method it will perhaps be well to consider in a critical way the methods used heretofore in studies of babyhood.

It is sufficient to say here that the method was a successful and practical way of obtaining data. Of the twenty-four mothers who undertook the study not one failed from lack of interest or cooperation to carry it through. During the two years 1,370 visits were made, 1,944 examinations were made by the observers, and a total of 4,181 records were obtained from the mothers.

METHODS COMMONLY USED IN STUDIES OF INFANTS

Psychological studies of infancy and early childhood have, in the main, employed three methods according to the aim of the study: first, the longitudinal method, if the aim of the study was to trace the course of development of a child over a long period; second, the cross-section method, if the aim was to set up standards of development for different age levels; and third, the training method, if the aim was to alter the course of development. The longitudinal method has been little used in studies of infancy. Oldest and most venerable from the standpoint of labor involved are the biographical studies that present a detailed account of the development of one or two children over a long period of time. The works of Preyer (25), Shinn (28), Moore (23), Major (22), and Fenton (11) amply illustrate this type of longitudinal study. (See Bibliography for references.)

The cross-section method has been employed in three types of studies. This method is used in obtaining norms for the development of any particular trait and in tracing the course of development of a trait from its earliest manifestations until it is completely established. Such studies require that the trait be observed in a large number of babies at closely spaced age levels. Jones's (17) study of the development of early behavior patterns illustrates the normative type of study, and Burnside's (8) study of locomotion represents an attempt to trace a trait throughout its course of development.

Inventories of the equipment of the infant at birth, such as those made by Watson and by Weiss and his students, take a cross-section survey of the child's behavior at the earliest possible age. A third application of the cross-section method is one in which the observer, after a comprehensive examination of large numbers of babies at widely spaced age levels, catalogues the traits that characterize the development at each age level. In this way norms are established, and a scale that can be used to determine the developmental levels of other babies is constructed. Gesell's (12) developmental schedules of the Yale Psycho-Clinic comprise such a study.

Although the training method has been used in many studies of older children, relatively few babies have been subjected to it in an experimental way. Watson's study of conditioning and Jones's study of unconditioning the fear response are examples of the conditioning method of training, and Hunter's delayed reaction experiment illustrates an application of the trial and error learning method to very young children.

The Longitudinal Method

Biographical studies. — Each method has, of course, certain advantages to recommend its use, and each has its own peculiar difficulties and disadvantages. The chief advantage of a biographical study is that, as a rule, daily notes are made on the child's development and behavior. Since the observer is usually a parent or a very near relative, the baby is under observation almost constantly day and night, and therefore very little of the infant's behavior escapes the adult's vigilant eye. Thus a large number of traits can be watched throughout their course of development. There is a further advantage that the traits are usually not tested for but are noticed only as they make their normal appearance. And finally there is the advantage that the baby is observed at home in his normal, everyday environment, so that he is absolutely undisturbed and unaware that he is attracting undue attention.

The difficulties and disadvantages of this method, however, are many. In the first place, there is no doubt that daily record-keeping is a long and laborious task, and it is small wonder that only a few studies of the kind have been made. Only a very few babies, usually one and never more than three, have been studied by each biographer. The observations recorded by these biographers cannot be combined to make a general picture of babyhood because, first, no two observers have recorded exactly the same things; second, most of the records are anecdotal, filled with tales of clever and remarkable tricks of the baby, which make interesting reading but which are very difficult to classify and put into general categories; third, such test situations as have been devised differ from baby to baby according to the whim and interest of the observer, and the method employed in the test is usually so obscurely described that it cannot be duplicated; and, finally, even observations of the same facts, such as age at sitting up, creeping, walking, and talking, recorded by all biographers are subject to the different criteria and interpretations of the various observers.

Even if it were possible to combine several biographical accounts, the composite biography could not be used as a standard for other children, because the children who have been the subjects of biographies form a highly selected group. Only the most interested and persistent of parents have gone to the trouble of keeping diaries of their babies, and only the superior ones have brought order out of the chaotic mass of data in the form of published accounts. It is rather likely, therefore, that such superior parents have superior children. Also the fact that the observers were mothers, fathers, or aunts of the babies probably made them subject to such errors as parental pride would lead them to make, in spite of their best efforts to guard against them.

The Cross-Section Method

Development of traits. — Many of the disadvantages of the biographical method are overcome in studies of the development of single traits. The observations are usually made by one person who examines each baby in the same laboratory room with the same apparatus and equipment and with a uniform procedure. Every possible condition is controlled, incentives are sometimes used to induce the baby to do the trick, and distractions are eliminated so far as possible. If a measuring scale can be devised for the trait it is measured; if not, each child's performance is at least described in the same terms according to the same observer's interpretation of it.

Nevertheless, this method, too, leaves much to be desired. Infants for such a study are usually obtained at baby welfare clinics; the very nature of this source makes for some selection of the babies. It is often difficult to get a large number of children at sufficiently close age levels, and it is usually impossible to get more than one or two retests on the same child. The examinations must be short, and consequently only a limited number of traits can be tested. The standardization of the test and the unusualness of the surroundings may rob the baby's behavior of its normal spontaneity and make his response a function of the experimental situations rather than of development. Finally, curves of development that are drawn up from observations on groups of different babies at succeeding age levels may represent in a true way the development of the trait in general, but they give no information as to the course of development of the trait in an individual baby.

Inventory at birth. — The birth inventory method

presents the same advantage of controlled conditions that characterizes the trait study. If the observer uses care in selecting the hospitals at which he does his observing, it is possible for him to get a large and comparatively random sample of babies for examination, since the majority of babies in most cities are born in hospitals. The birth inventory, however useful it may be, is still limited to a very short age range and to the observation of a few traits. Weiss's method of continuous observation over a two-week period has the special disadvantage that the observers have to relieve each other in long day and night vigils and that after several hours of watching and recording the baby's slightest stir the observers no doubt become both fatigued and bored.

Normative summary. — The chief advantage of the normative summary, over and above the advantages of control of conditions and standardization of method that have been mentioned above, is that this method allows the observer to test for a large number of traits and thereby enables him to get a summary of the baby's general level of ability at any age. Babies for most studies of this nature are obtained through the interest and cooperation of the mother, and this may serve as a selecting factor. Neither the general course of development nor the rate of progress of an individual child can be studied by this method. Finally, the difficulties of motivating a baby in a test situation are very great. It is probable that chance factors have greater weight in determining the test score for a baby than for an older child or for an adult, and consequently that a verdict as to the developmental age of a baby can be pronounced from a single test with much less surety.

The Training Method

The same advantage of controlled conditions holds for training studies. The difficulty that besets this method in particular is that only in homes, in orphanages, or in day nurseries is it possible for the observer to get the day-to-day contact that is necessary for training the baby. Added to this is the difficulty that there are practically no incentives that can be used in training. Human sympathy precludes the use of pain or punishment in training the baby, and the physical welfare of the baby makes hunger an unwise motive. Finally, the current theory that the child is more impressionable at early than at later ages and that early experiences leave a mark never to be effaced may well make an experimenter pause before he launches upon a course of training or conditioning.

THE PRESENT STUDY

Since the objective was to make a comprehensive and intensive study of both physical growth and psychological development, the longitudinal method was decided upon for use in this study. The plan was to follow the development of twenty-five babies throughout a two-year period by making repeated examinations at frequent intervals. As it has worked out the study has actually been the extension of the biographical method of child study to include many babies instead of one.

Such a method of study is long and laborious. It is obviously impossible to condense the study into a short period of time, for a two-year study on the same babies demands no less than twenty-four successive months of observation. The wastefulness of this method makes it impractical for use when only general trends of development are sought, and the impossibility of studying large groups by this method makes it useless for establishing norms. Nevertheless, it is the only method that can be used for tracing the course of developmental processes in detail and for obtaining information on habits and on traits of personality that persist over long periods of time.

The aims of the study were: (1) to trace the course of development of mental and motor processes over a two-year period in a group of twenty-five babies; (2) to discover whether personality traits and habits are transitory or constant during the first two years; (3) to attempt to get an integrated picture of the development and of the behavior traits of each child; and (4) to have such physical, anthropometric, and psychological data on each baby that each might be used to supplement and explain the results of the other.

The Method in General

Source of the babies for study. — Perhaps the most obvious difficulty of all the methods of infant study discussed above is that of finding babies for study. Nowhere in modern society do infants occur in large, unselected groups, all growing up under uniform care. Orphanages and day nurseries have been cited above as sources of large groups of babies, but these babies in general come from the lower strata of society. The nursery school program is gradually extending the school age downward so that groups of very young children are now available for study. But the vast majority of babies under two years are to be found in homes, growing up under parental care, and apart from its desirability or undesirability home care is a régime that probably will outlast many of our modern institutions.

Consequently, if a study of babyhood is to have

either practical or theoretical importance, babies chosen for the study should be living in homes under the care of their parents. Furthermore, the modern baby is not fetched and carried from place to place, and the length of the proposed study and the frequency of the examinations certainly made it impossible for the mother to bring the baby to the laboratory to be studied. The only alternative was for the observers to go to the homes for each examination. Hence all observations and tests were made with the baby in his normal habitat, his mother either being present or within earshot.

The observers. — All observations were made jointly by two women, B and S. The former, a pediatrician, was in charge of the physical and anthropometric examinations. S, a psychologist, devised and directed the program of psychological tests. The cooperation of the two investigators made it possible to take more complete observations and to proceed with the work at a more rapid pace than if each had worked alone.

Contact with the mothers. — Since the babies were to be observed each day during the hospital period as well as at weekly intervals in the home, it was necessary to make contact with the mother before the baby was born and to get her consent to the study. Most of the contacts with the mothers were made through obstetricians who were interested in the project. Letters were sent by the obstetricians to their patients, and upon favorable replies the two investigators called on the expectant mothers and set forth their plans. It was explained that many of the present standards of physical and mental development had been based on children living in institutions but that they were not adequate for judging infants who were living at home under modern nutritional care. For this reason it was desirable to collect material on physical and mental growth from a group of healthy babies who were growing up in homes under present-day medical care. The mother was told that the examiners would call once a week for a thirty-minute examination of the baby, and that she would be asked to keep a daily record of the baby's weight, his feeding, and his sleeping and to note items of development and behavior that she observed during the day.

The mother was to be furnished with an accurate scale for weighing the baby and with a wall thermometer to hang near the crib. It was made clear to her that the examiners would not take the responsibility of the baby's medical care other than to point out symptoms of illness if she should fail to see them and to advise her to consult her regular pediatrician.

Selection of the babies. — At the outset it was planned to take babies from the second, third, and fourth parturitions only. The reason for the discrimination against first babies was, on the physical side, that first babies are on the average somewhat smaller than children born later, and, on the psychological side, that first babies are usually more of an event in the household, cause much more upset in the family routine, and are likely to be hovered over with more anxious care than later babies. The mother who has watched one child through infancy is perhaps more competent to observe and record the behavior of another baby. However, it was impractical to adhere to the rule of excluding first babies, and a few were taken. In the final group three babies were first-born, thirteen were second-born, seven were third-born, and four were fourth-born. At first it was planned to restrict the study to a residential district near the University, but since the examiners were unable to make contact with enough mothers in this district to furnish the required number of babies, the study was extended to include the whole city.

No attempt was made to make the group of twenty-five babies a representative sampling of the population. Since the cooperation of intelligent and interested mothers was of chief importance in carrying out the study, it was deemed best not to penetrate to families of low economic status. The fathers of the babies studied included lawyers, physicians, ministers, salesmen, college professors, retail merchants, a clerk, a machinist, skilled tradesmen, a civil engineer, and business managers of local firms. A classification of the occupations of the fathers according to the occupational scale in use at the Minnesota Institute of Child Welfare gave the following results.

Occupational Group	Fathers of Babies Studied		Total Population
	No. of Cases	Per Cent	in Per Cent
Professional	9	37.5	5.4
Managerial	3	12.5	6.3
Salesmen and dealers	12	50.0	37.5

It is obvious that these babies represent a highly selected group. The entire number is drawn from the three upper occupational classes, and the three lower classes, which comprise a total of 50.8 per cent of the population, are entirely unrepresented. Nevertheless, the group is less selected than are the babies of biographical studies and probably is as representative of the general population as are samplings drawn from welfare clinics, since the patients of free clinics would come largely from the three lower occupational groups.

Several of the mothers had a college education, and

some of them had been employed as teachers, stenographers, and telephone operators before marriage. Fourteen of the mothers each had one full-time maid; the remaining eleven mothers did all of their own housework. All of them had enough leisure and interest in their babies to undertake the study and to carry it through.

Most of the babies were born in the autumn. The first two, on whom incomplete preliminary data were collected, were born in July. Of the remainder, three were born in September, nine in October, and thirteen in November. Whatever effect season may have had on the babies' development was the same for all. The fact that all babies went through the winter first may have had some slight influence on their behavior development, since spring and summer babies are less completely bundled in clothing during the day and are more often put on the floor and given opportunities for creeping.[1]

Intervals of testing. — Originally it was planned to examine the babies only at monthly intervals. But it was immediately apparent that the infant became fatigued by a long examination and that short examinations repeated at frequent intervals yielded much more complete and dependable data. Because of the rapid neonatal changes the babies were observed daily during the first week and every other day during the second week. After the hospital period the babies were examined at weekly intervals during the first year and biweekly during the second year.

Number of babies studied. — Practically all the mothers who were interested enough to ask for an interview agreed to come into the study. There were twenty-seven

[1] A condensed family history of each baby is to be found under *Dramatis Personae*, Appendix 6.

babies at the start of the experiment. One had to be operated on for pyloric stenosis at the age of one month, and although his recovery was rapid and complete the mother did not feel equal to assuming the obligation of the study after his illness. One family moved from town when the infant was 18 weeks old, and two others moved away when the babies were 40 weeks old. Complete records for the entire first year were obtained on twenty-four babies. At the end of the first year one mother discontinued the study; early in the second year one baby died; two records were discontinued because the families moved from the city, and large gaps occurred in some of the babies' records during the second summer, when several families left the city for vacations. For twenty of the twenty-five cases records are reasonably complete to 18 months, and for sixteen they are complete to 2 years.

The Examining Technique

Seriatim records collected on each baby throughout the entire period included: (1) anthropometric measurements at regular intervals; (2) records of the baby's health, nutrition, and general physical well-being, and a summary of illnesses; (3) records of motor coordination, both gross and fine; (4) records of sensory development; (5) notes on development of speech; (6) notes as to interest in objects, choice of toys, and so forth; and (7) notes on behavior and personality traits that appeared as a by-product of the examination.

There were two requirements that limited the choice of tests: first, the tests must not disturb the mother; and, secondly, the equipment must be simple and portable. For this study to go forward at all it was necessary above everything else to keep the interest and cooperation of the mothers. This fact limited the investigators somewhat in their choice of tests. The tests had to be of such a nature that they disturbed neither mother nor baby. They had to be short enough not to tire the baby, and the apparatus and instruments used had to be simple, light, and of such nature that they could be cleaned and sterilized easily.

The investigators traveled by automobile to all parts of Minneapolis and examined from six to ten babies a day. Equipment had to be limited, therefore, to a few essentials that could be carried about and easily packed and unpacked. About forty pounds of luggage was carried, but the major pieces of equipment, such as cribs, examining tables, crawling rugs, and high chairs, had to be furnished in the home. This made it impossible to standardize the equipment; the examiners merely used whatever the mother had.

Medical and anthropometric equipment was indispensable, and since carrying space was at a premium, the calipers, stethoscope, and tape measures were made to serve double duty — as medical instruments and as standardized toys for the babies. A special kit was made to hold the blood pressure apparatus, cloth for fontanelle tracing, a bag of wooden blocks, a cup, a box of fabrics, a bottle of alcohol for cleaning instruments, and two filing spaces, one for blank records and one for used records. A tray contained a pair of straight calipers, a pair of bow calipers, tape measures, tongue blades, pencils, a stop watch, a hand ball, a harmonica, paper clips, rubber bands, a roll of paper for taking footprints, picture books, and other simple toys. After the examination of each baby the instruments were cleaned with alcohol, and at the end of the day's examination the kit was taken into the laboratory and cleaned thoroughly.

This kit weighed about twenty-five pounds. A measuring board especially constructed for the purpose was also carried. Later in the experiment a metal stand for a photographer's screen, the frame of which was strung with wires to make a 1½-inch wire network, was added to the equipment.

This apparatus was compact enough to be carried in and out of the houses, to be set up and torn down and packed promptly, and on cold days to be warmed to room temperature in a few minutes. More elaborate set-ups and better standardized major equipment, particularly examining tables, would have been desirable but would not have been practicable in an experiment of this kind.

INFANT STUDY EXAMINATION SCHEDULE

First Year

AGE	TYPE OF EXAMINATION
1 day	Anthropometric and brief physical
2–6 days	Daily hospital, physical and psychological
7 days	Anthropometric
9, 11, 13 days	Daily hospital, physical and psychological
14 days	Anthropometric
3 weeks	Weekly physical and psychological
4 weeks	Anthropometric
5 weeks	Weekly physical and psychological
6 weeks	Anthropometric
7 weeks	Weekly physical and psychological
8 weeks	Anthropometric
9–11 weeks	Weekly physical and psychological
12 weeks	Anthropometric
13 weeks	Tests of Development
14 weeks	Tests of Development, short physical
15 weeks	Tests of Development
16 weeks	Anthropometric and physical
17 weeks	Developmental schedule, Yale Psycho-Clinic, 4 months
18 weeks	Tests of Development, short physical
19 weeks	Tests of Development
20 weeks	Anthropometric and physical
21–23 weeks	Tests of Development

AGE	TYPE OF EXAMINATION
24 weeks	Anthropometric and physical
25 weeks	Choice Test I
26 weeks	Developmental schedule, Yale Psycho-Clinic, 6 months
27 weeks	Choice Test I
28 weeks	Anthropometric and physical
29 weeks	Choice Test I
30–31 weeks	Choice Test II
32 weeks	Anthropometric and physical
33 weeks	Color Choice Test
34 weeks	Form Choice Test
35 weeks	Textile Choice Test
36 weeks	Anthropometric and physical
37 weeks	Box Test
38 weeks	Tests of Development. Retest after lapse of 15 weeks. Baby allowed to examine contents of instrument case for five minutes
39 weeks	Developmental schedule, Yale Psycho-Clinic, 9 months
40 weeks	Anthropometric and physical
41 weeks	Box Test
42 weeks	Picture and Perfume Test
43 weeks	Party
44 weeks	Anthropometric and physical
45 weeks	Box Test
46 weeks	Color Choice Test
47 weeks	Form Choice Test
48 weeks	Anthropometric and physical
49 weeks	Box Test
50 weeks	Picture and Perfume Test
51 weeks	Developmental schedule, Yale Psycho-Clinic, 12 months
52 weeks	Anthropometric and physical
SECOND YEAR	
54–74 weeks (4-week intervals)	Infant Study Psychological Test
78 weeks	Minnesota Preschool Test
78–102 weeks (4-week intervals)	Infant Study Psychological Test
104 weeks	Minnesota Preschool Test
56–104 weeks (4-week intervals)	Anthropometric and physical

Explanation of the schedule. — On the day after the mother went home from the hospital the investigators called at the home to deliver the scale and usually saw the baby for a moment. In most cases the mothers left the hospital on the 13th or 14th day. In case the mother left earlier, the examiners made an effort to call on the 12th or 13th day in addition to the 14th in order to make the records uniform with those of babies who remained in the hospital two weeks. In case an extra call at the home could not be made, the two-week physical rather than the anthropometric test was omitted. It was not possible to do both of these tests on the same day, because the long examination fatigued the baby.

It will be noted that in scheduling anthropometric measurements the lunar month of four weeks rather than the calendar month was followed. This was done in order to avoid the inequality of months as marked by the birth date. The arrangement of the tests of behavior and development follows no preconceived plan, and the order may not seem particularly logical. From inspecting the schedule one infers that tests of behavior and development were given on whatever weeks remained after the anthropometric and the Yale Psychological tests had been scheduled. After the 6th month psychological tests were varied frequently in order to fit the rapid development of the baby's abilities and interests. Choice Tests I and II were given from the 25th through the 31st week. Color and form choice tests were introduced twice, and the box test four times at four-week intervals during the remainder of the year. At the 38th week a retest with the test of development was carried out in order to contrast the behavior of the baby at this age with his behavior on the same test 15 weeks earlier. Time did not permit retests with the fabric tests.

In devising the psychological tests an effort was made to include items that would be of interest to the baby and would call forth many different types of reactions from him. No contention is made that the tests were properly placed at the various age levels or that they were especially devised to bring out the child's most advanced behavior at each age. Subsequent analysis has shown that some of the tests might profitably have been started at an earlier age and that others might have continued to a later age than originally used. All the tests had interest value for the babies, and all yielded useful data.

Division of work by the experimenters. — At the outset of the experiment it was decided that one of the investigators should do all the handling of the infant, the manipulating of the instruments, and the administering of the tests, and that the other should do all the note-taking. This seemed desirable for the reason that the baby would be subject to only one "type" of handling throughout the experiment and that the note-taking would be subject to the errors, omissions, and abbreviations of only one person. Since the pediatrician had to handle the baby for the physical examination and since she already was skilled in the technique of anthropometric measurement, it was agreed that she take charge of the baby and that the psychologist take her dictation and observe and record the behavior of the infant. Throughout this report the pediatrician will be referred to as Experimenter B and the psychologist as Experimenter S.

Examining room. — For the hospital examinations the investigators were allowed to work at the tables on which the babies were bathed. In some cases this was in the nursery where the babies slept, and in others it was located in an adjoining room. Usually there were one or two nurses working in the same room, and in some hospitals where the nursery was crowded the examining room was both congested and noisy. In all cases the nurses were courteous and helpful, and the examiners endeavored to keep out of the way and to interfere with hospital routine as little as possible.

In the home the examination was done in whatever room the mother saw fit to use. Many preferred that the examiners work in the bathroom on a canvas bath table. The bathroom was most often used for the anthropometric measurements, during which the baby was completely undressed, because as a rule it could be warmed more quickly than the larger rooms. In other homes the examination was done on the kitchen table. This was the most convenient place to work since there was more space for spreading out instruments. In some homes a bedroom was used, the bed serving as a table for the examination. As the children grew older and were promoted to high-chair tests and to sitting on the floor, the examinations were often conducted in the living room, the nursery, occasionally in a sunroom, or out-of-doors on the lawn. A note of the examining quarters was made on the later records when it was thought that surroundings might present distracting stimuli for the baby.

Audience. — Naturally the mothers were both concerned for the babies' welfare and interested in their reactions to the tests. Since it was necessary above all else to keep the mothers' interest and confidence, they were invited to watch the examination if they cared to but were assured that it was not necessary for them to remain in the room if they wished to be busy elsewhere. Most of the mothers did watch the early examinations, but after the first few weeks they became used to the procedure and, confident that the baby was in safe hands, often left the room. Other small children in the family frequently watched the examination and occasionally had to be kept from interfering with it. Neighbors or callers sometimes asked to see the examination, and now and then a grandmother or a father was present. When any person other than the investigators was present there was always more or less conversation. The mother often took this opportunity to report to interested listeners all the ups and downs of the baby's week and to ask advice on such problems as whether the baby's room was kept warm enough, how to prevent thumb-sucking, and the like. If callers were present the examiners merely as a matter of courtesy usually explained very briefly the nature of the study and the reason for the choice of tests. And if young children were around the examiners had to pay some attention to their childish comments or keep them occupied with some harmless instrument from the examining kit.

After such a description of the general setting in which the experiments were made one hardly needs to add that the investigators made almost no effort to keep out of the picture themselves. They conversed only when it was necessary; they looked at the baby, smiled at him now and then, and occasionally in later tests spoke to him in tones of praise or encouragement. They stood where they could observe and be observed by the baby; their position was constant for a single examination but varied slightly from baby to baby and from examination to examination. The idea of setting up screens behind which the experimenters could work unobserved by the baby was abandoned because it would have involved the carrying about and setting up of too much apparatus. Furthermore, for the examiners to have hidden themselves and remained silent while members of the family circulated about freely and talked to the baby would have been to strain at gnats and swallow camels.

An examination under such circumstances certainly leaves much to be desired in the way of controlling conditions. On the other hand, it meets the criticism so often made of laboratory experiments that the strangeness of the situation and the artificiality of the conditions rob the baby of naturalness and spontaneity of response. Most laboratory observers, therefore, strive to duplicate home conditions and to put the baby at his ease before starting the examination. In this experiment the investigators had actual home conditions for each baby. Playing with the baby before starting the examinations was usually unnecessary, since the experimenters saw the baby so often that they were as familiar to him as grandmothers or aunts, and their arrival was usually greeted with smiles and later with shouts of recognition. In the second year more than one child came to the door and ran back to mother calling, "Mamma, Doctor's come."

Anthropometric measurements in detail. — From the anthropometric measurements valuable behavior data were obtained. Although they are not really classified with the psychological tests, they formed an important part of the examining scheme. The procedures used in this examination were similar to those in the psychological tests; consequently, this detailed description is given here to familiarize the reader with the examining routine.

The record form for the anthropometric examination consisted of a four-page folder (see Appendix 1). Along the margin were printed the names of the measurements taken, and a space opposite was left for recording the measure in centimeters. The rest of the sheet was divided into convenient spaces with appropriate headings at the top for checking the child's behavior during each measurement. Space was provided at the top of the first page for recording the name of the child, the date, the hour of examination, the birth date, and the baby's age in weeks. On the fourth page of the folder there was space for a summary of the baby's behavior during the examination. The reflexes were also recorded along with the measures. Logically they are a part of the physical examination, but to include them there made that examination too long for the very young infant.

The order in which the measures are arranged on the blank is one in which all the measures involving manipulation of the head come first, measurements of the arms and trunk next, and measures of the legs last. The blanks were printed in this order rather than in the more convenient order of circumferences, bilateral diameters, anterior-posterior diameters, and lengths because, as a result of the first few examinations, it seemed best to expose only one section of the baby's body at a time. Later it was discovered that this order entailed considerably more manipulation of the infant and was more likely to call forth a protest than the latter order, so during most of the experiment the order followed was circumferences, diameters, lengths. As the babies reached the rolling and crawling stage B often had to modify the order again to fit in with the baby's activities, and the measuring process almost became a game of catch-as-catch-can between B and the baby with the odds in favor of the baby.

The baby was laid upon a table and was restricted as little as possible during the measuring. For the circumferences and bilateral diameters the baby was laid on his back. The anterior-posterior diameters and lengths involved placing the baby on his right side and on his left, since measurements of both sides of the body had to be taken. The reflexes were done after all the measurements except the final lengths were taken. In doing the biceps, triceps, and knee jerk B tapped the tendon ten times in succession or until the jerk was elicited. The number of the tap at which the jerk occurred was recorded in the space, and if no jerk occurred in ten trials a zero was recorded. The Babinski stimulus was given five times on each foot by B's scratching the sole of the baby's foot slightly with her index fingernail. The partial responses were checked under extension of great toe, fan of other toes, jerk of foot, or plantar response, and jerk of opposite. Indeterminate responses were described as well as possible. The crown-rump and crown-heel measurements were reserved till the very last of the examination, because the babies usually fussed at these measures. The baby was placed on a special measuring board having a stationary headboard and a sliding footboard. B held the baby's head and trunk gently in place while S straightened the baby's knee, slid the footboard up till it touched the soles of his feet, and read the scale.

The complete set of measurements and reflexes required about twenty minutes under ordinary circumstances. Under very favorable conditions with the baby quiet and not interfering the time was often reduced to fifteen minutes. When the baby interfered by catching instruments or playing with toys the examination lengthened out to twenty-five minutes. Now and then the baby had to be picked up and quieted for a moment, and often its diaper had to be changed during the examination. If the baby lay quietly and watched without fussing or interfering, no effort was made to divert him. Although it sometimes happened that the baby was no more active than if he had been an inanimate object, it more frequently happened that he was an interested spectator or participator in the measuring, and at those times B or S had to entertain him as well as measure and record his behavior. At the early ages a tape measure or toy was dangled before him to hold his attention. Sometimes the mother helped by holding a toy or patting the baby and talking to him in soothing tones. After the baby began to reach for objects he was given a tape or a bell to keep his busy fingers away from B's instruments. B dictated the measures in a low voice to S, who stood near and recorded the measures and at the same time watched and recorded by check marks or by abbreviated phrases the behavior of the infant during the measure. It was impossible, of course, to get everything the baby did on paper even in the early weeks when his range of activity was limited, and it became increasingly more difficult to do so as the baby's behavior became more complex. The crying column, however, was carefully checked throughout the experiment. Eye, arm, and leg movements were recorded in the early months. After 5 or 6 months, however, these finer categories were ignored and such notes as "catches B's caliper," "plays with Doctor's hair," "takes tape and chews it," "reaches for bell and rings it vigorously," were made opposite the general section of measures in which they occurred.

Mothers' records. — The mothers were furnished with printed forms for keeping daily records of the child's weight, feedings, daily habits, signs of development, and daily conduct. The mother laid aside each day's record as it was completed, and the week's quota were collected by the investigators at their weekly visit.

Three different forms were made out for the mothers'

records (see Appendixes 2, 3, 4, and 5): the first was used for the period from 2 to 12 weeks, the second for the period from 12 to 32 weeks, and the third from 32 to 52 weeks. The identification data called for on each record included the baby's name, the date, the baby's birth date, his age in days or weeks, and his weight. As a safeguard against mixing the blanks of different babies a key number in red was put on all the sheets in the record pad for each baby. This made it possible to salvage any records from which the mother had omitted the baby's name.

Form I allowed space for a complete feeding record. In a wide column at the left margin the items to be noted at the feeding time were listed. The width of the page was divided into six columns, and each column was assigned to one of the six daily feeding periods. In these columns the mother checked or wrote in the behavior at each nursing. This record was more detailed than necessary, since the baby's nursing was usually undisturbed. Although the mothers were not requested to weigh the babies before and after nursing to determine the amount taken, many of them did it for their own information, and when they did so they recorded the amount taken. Below the nursing record was space for noting the baby's daily habits, such as bowel movements, sleeping, and crying spells. In order that the record might show roughly the time of day at which such events occurred, the six columns denoting feeding time were extended down into the space allotted to habits, and the mother then checked these occurrences in the appropriate column to indicate after which feeding period the event took place. A bowel movement that occurred between the 10:00 A.M. and the 2:00 P.M. feeding period, for example, would be checked in the second column.

The rest of the page was devoted to signs of development, which were briefly described and which were to be checked by the mother. Space was left for her to add notes or to qualify or amplify any of the descriptive terms. A space at the bottom of the sheet gave room for the mother to summarize on a 5-point scale the general conduct of the baby for the day, and there was another space for her to check any physical disturbances that she had noted.

On the reverse side of the sheet were blanks for describing possible frights, anger, accidents, signs of affection, or any unusual happening or upsets in the family schedule.

In Form II the feeding and habit records were condensed somewhat to allow more space for developmental items and more space for the mother to write additional items. It called for essentially the same information, however, as did Form I. The reverse side was the same as that of Form I.

Forms I and II were for daily records. As the child grew older and as his rate of development slowed down, his daily routine became very well established so that a weekly record was adequate for catching changes in the habit schedule and new signs of development. This weekly record consisted of a four-page folder. Page 1 was devoted to a summary of the regular feeding schedule and the regular habit schedule with additional space on which the mother could record any departures from the daily schedule, the baby's weight, and a summary of his conduct for each day. An additional column contained a list of developmental items that pertained particularly to the baby's eating and personal habits. Page 2 was given over to developmental items concerning gross motor control, comprehension of language, and the use of sounds as speech. The developmental items on page 3 were concerned with the development of the senses, fine motor control, play reactions, and personality reactions. The last page was the same as that for Forms I and II, with additional space for describing the methods used and the success of the mother in training the child for bowel movements and in breaking him of thumb-sucking.

At a casual glance these record blanks look formidable. It is obvious, however, that no baby did all the things listed on any one day and that no mother had to check every item every day. Most of the blanks could be filled simply by checking a few items, and in a short time the mothers became familiar enough with the records so that they did not need to read through the entire list of items in order to check the record for a single day. No estimate can be made of the time spent by the mothers in keeping these records. Suffice it to say that some records were kept by all the mothers, and complete records were kept for twenty of the twenty-five babies throughout the first year. For those who are skeptical as to the value of these records it may be worth while to state here a few facts that will be discussed more fully later. Most mothers checked the records with great care; many wrote additional records and notes on the blanks; two mothers of twins each kept two daily records instead of one; mothers in general did not tend to overstate the ability of babies; in almost no instance where the mother recorded a precocious or amusing trick on the part of the child did the investigators fail to verify her record at their next visit.

Criticism of the Present Study

Many of the difficulties that assail other methods of studying developing infants are obviated by the methods used in this investigation, and many of the criticisms that can be directed against other studies are either met or offset in this work. This study is most similar to the biographical studies in that it traces the development of traits in individual children over long periods of time and under home conditions. It meets the chief objections to the biographical studies on the following points:

1. From twenty to twenty-five babies were observed, as compared to the observations of one, two, or three children by the biographers.

2. The babies varied over a much wider range in socio-economic status and probably in intelligence than the babies in the biographical studies.

3. The records were made comparable from baby to baby since: (a) The same tests at the same age were made on each baby, and the facts observed were recorded in the same terms. In essential features the examinations did not vary from one baby to another. (b) The recording was done by checking items made out in advance or by making brief descriptions of the baby's behavior in set phrases. Although anecdotes were collected to supplement the accounts, they were not relied upon for the bulk of the material. (c) The observations and interpretations were subject to the errors and omissions of only one recorder, and such errors would tend to affect all records alike. (d) Since the investigators were neither parents nor relatives but impartial observers and since the observations of the mother were checked each week by the observers, there is very little likelihood that the baby's performance was overstated.

The study presents many of the advantages of laboratory studies. The procedure was standard, the observers were the same, and a fairly large and constant number of babies were examined at each age. To be sure, this study lacked the elaborate apparatus and the perfect control of conditions that laboratory examinations make possible. It seems likely, however, that bare white walls, soundproof rooms, constant temperature, tables and equipment of regulation size and design are relatively unimportant in getting the baby to watch moving objects, smile, reach for and manipulate toys, sit alone, or walk. At any rate, they are much less important than having the baby completely at his ease in a familiar and friendly environment. The chances are good that, with length of examinations, nature and sequence of tests, age of administering tests, and familiarity of home setting constant for all babies, the essential features of the examinations were controlled.

The methods of any study can be evaluated only in the light of the problems the experimenter sets out to solve. The problems in this study were those of tracing the course and rate of development of many traits both in the group and in the individual, of observing the nature and constancy of personality traits, of studying the interrelation and the integration of traits in the group and in the individual, and of obtaining parallel physical development. Features of this method that recommend it above other methods are:

1. Observations on the same babies were taken over a long period of time.

2. During the examination the baby was at ease in the home situation.

3. The frequency of examinations allowed for observing a larger number of traits and for checking previous observations the following week.

4. The range of babies, although somewhat limited, was confined neither to the upper nor to the lower strata of the socio-economic scale.

5. The apparatus and procedure were so simple and so nearly duplicated the baby's own toys and daily experiences that his performance was natural and spontaneous rather than a function of the test. If any data on babies are uncorrupted by the methods of testing, these data should be so.

6. The simplicity and usualness of the tests made it unlikely that they would influence the baby's normal course of development. An effort was made to devise situations that would call forth in the course of the thirty-minute observation most of the acts that the baby had done spontaneously during the preceding week.

The study was by no means perfect. The two most salient objections to it are that the cases were too few to establish norms of development and that the weekly examinations were too infrequent to attempt training experiments. But there are other less laborious and less time-consuming methods of collecting data for those purposes. For tracing the course of development of modern babies in their native haunts and for making detailed observations of each baby's idiosyncracies repeated examination in the home is not only the best but the only possible method.

CHAPTER II

PURPOSE AND METHODS OF STUDYING LOCOMOTOR DEVELOPMENT

The purposes of the study of motor development as well as the aim of the study as a whole were: (1) to trace the course of motor development in its many phases from birth to the age of walking alone; (2) to discover interrelations of various phases of motor development and their relation to anatomical and physical development; (3) to study individual differences in the rate of motor development; and (4) to consider theoretical implications of motor development.

The data on motor development came from three sources: motor tests given by the observers as a regular part of each psychological examination, daily record sheets kept by the mothers, and "incidental items," the name given to all reactions that occurred spontaneously during the examination.

Motor Tests

All the motor tests were simple and followed the same general plan. Since they usually involved more manipulation of the baby than did tests of reaching and playing with toys and since manipulation was more likely to upset the baby, the motor tests were deferred till the end of the examination. This order was not adopted until the 13th week of examination. During the early weeks the babies were usually found lying in their cribs, and the motor tests were done in the early part of the examination as a means of getting their interest and attention.

Creeping. — One simple test for creeping was used throughout the entire first year. The baby was placed on his stomach on a flat surface, a table or the floor, and observed in that position for one minute. From the 13th week on a bell was rung and placed just out of reach and directly in front of the baby. This bell was a favorite toy with all the babies and was an adequate incentive to creeping. The reactions of the baby in this posture were consistently recorded, reactions such as turning the head, lifting the head and chest, pushing with the feet or toes, drawing up the knees in a frog-like position, kicking the legs and waving the arms as if swimming, turning or pivoting so that the head pointed a different direction, rolling onto the side or back, making progress by any means whatever, moving backward, pushing to a sitting posture, and hitching or creeping on all fours.

No feasible method could be devised for measuring the baby's skill at these performances, although three methods were tried. One method consisted in noting the promptness of the baby in making a reaction by means of recording the number of seconds that elapsed before he lifted his head, rolled, or crept as the case might be. Another method was to record the length of time he persisted in the reaction, and the third was an attempt to measure the distance traversed by the baby in the one-minute interval. None of these methods was useful in the end. The promptness of the baby's adjustment depended as often upon his interest as upon his skill; his persistence depended largely upon how quickly he obtained the bell, for obviously his reaching and wiggling stopped the moment he got the toy, and the value of the situation as a test of creeping was over. Finally, the distance he traversed was frequently backward and usually circuitous, so that measurement would have meant very little. The account of creeping was, therefore, wholly descriptive rather than quantitative.

Rolling. — The baby's ability to roll was tested by placing him for one minute on his back. During the early weeks he was observed without any toy or incentive for rolling, but he was stimulated to watch a moving object and to reach for it. From 6 months on the bell was rung and placed on the baby's right at his shoulder level and just beyond the reach of his right hand. In order to get the bell it was necessary for the baby to hitch over or to roll. The records for this test were also limited to descriptive accounts.

Head control. — Throughout the early weeks the investigators searched for a simple and effective test of the baby's ability to hold his head erect. A most promising method was at last hit upon. It consisted in grasping the baby's wrists when he was lying on his back and pulling him to a sitting posture. Babies who had achieved a fair degree of head control tensed their neck muscles so that the head remained in the body line while they were being pulled up. Those in whom head control was not yet established allowed their heads to drop back at an angle. Unfortunately this test of head control was discovered too late for consistent records to be taken on all the babies.

Sitting on lap. — The first test of sitting was made with the baby seated on the examiner's lap, his back leaning against her bosom. She gave him support by placing her hands on each side of his chest. Five gradations of support were given in this way according to whether Examiner B placed her hands just under the baby's arms, at his midribs, at his lower ribs, at his hips, or whether he sat with no support at all except that given by the cupping of the examiner's lap and by the baby's leaning against her. Head control in this posture was estimated by the observer as none, partial, or complete, and was the only descriptive term used other than those indicating at what point B's hands supported the baby.

Tensing muscles for being lifted. — This test was made by B's noting whether the baby tensed his muscles to adjust for being lifted when she slipped her hands beneath his shoulders for lifting him.

Sitting alone. — The test of sitting alone was made with the baby seated on the floor with legs wide apart for support. The bell was put on the floor directly in front and within easy reach. The baby usually took the bell and played with it throughout the test. Time was used as a measure of proficiency in this test. If the baby sat alone as long as one minute, it was considered that sitting alone was established. If he fell, the length of time he sat before falling was taken as the measure of his skill. If the baby fell before one minute elapsed, he was given two other trials at sitting. The one-minute interval proved an excellent criterion for the skill of sitting alone. Usually if the baby fell in less than one minute at the first trial he fell in almost the same time at the second and third trials, whereas if he maintained his balance for sixty seconds he usually sat much longer.

Standing with help. —The earliest test of standing was made by holding the baby erect with support under his armpits and with his feet touching the table or the floor. His attempts at alternate stepping or prancing and his efforts to straighten his knee and hip joints and to bear some weight on his feet were noted. This test was supplanted after the 17th week by the walking test.

Pulling to standing position by means of furniture. — For this test the baby was seated on the floor in front of a davenport or chair. The faithful bell was rung and set on top of the chair to tempt the baby to climb. The observer recorded whether the baby got to his knees and whether he pulled himself completely to the standing posture. The time required to make these adjustments was also recorded but was found to be valueless for the reasons already mentioned. The test continued for a one-minute interval.

Standing by furniture. — If the baby rose to the standing posture during the one-minute interval, he was allowed to stand for one minute longer; if he fell or sat down, the number of seconds he stood was recorded. The baby who was unable to lift himself to the standing posture during the first minute was placed in a standing posture by the chair and allowed to stand for one minute. Three trials were given as in the sitting test in case he fell before the end of the minute. The latter two tests were begun when the baby was 37 weeks old.

Walking. — The walking test, which was begun in the 5th month and carried throughout the remainder of the two years, will be described in a later chapter.

Summary of the tests. — All motor tests except those for walking were discontinued at the end of the first year, since all the skills represented were fully developed in all the babies by that age. No new motor tests were undertaken in the second year, and walking alone represents the highest type of motor skill studied. More advanced skills were frequently observed and will be discussed under motor play.

Signs of Motor Development Recorded by Mothers

Items recorded. — A large number of items on locomotor development were included in the list of developmental traits on the mothers' records. On the earliest records, which were used daily from 3 to 12 weeks, the items were:

Turning from side to back or stomach
Turning from stomach to back or back to stomach
Rolling completely from back to back or stomach to stomach
Lifting head when on stomach, chin up
Lifting head when on stomach, chest up
Tensing muscles for being lifted

On the second daily record sheet, which was used when the babies were between 13 and 32 weeks, the items on lifting the head and tensing the muscles were omitted, those on turning and rolling were retained, and the following items were added:

Sitting when propped with pillows
Pushing self to sitting posture in crib
Sitting alone. How long? ....
Pushing with toes when lying on stomach
Creeping or hitching
Pushing feet against lap when held erect, feet touching
Making stepping movements when held with feet touching table
Pulling self to standing posture in crib
Standing holding to furniture
Walking holding to furniture
Standing alone
Walking alone

This list was so long and complete that many of the reactions were not established before the 32nd week. All the items on rolling, creeping, standing, and walking had to be repeated in the weekly record blank that was used from 32 to 52 weeks. New items were:

Rolling completely two or three times in succession
Going on all fours
Walking, pushing furniture in front
Walking alone. How many steps? . . . .
Climbing upstairs on all fours
Climbing downstairs
Climbing on stools or chairs
Climbing off stools or chairs
Propelling kiddy-car
Rocking in rocking chairs
Bouncing in baby swing
Bouncing on stuffed chairs
Bouncing or dancing to music

Space was provided for the mother to describe other activities and tricks of the baby as well as his method of crawling or creeping.

Consistency of checking.—The mothers' records, it will be remembered, included a complete feeding record and called for daily weights and many other physical items as well as for developmental data. Some mothers filled out one part more completely than another according to their own interests and their ideas as to which were more important. In general the weight record, feeding chart, and statement of the baby's health took precedence over the developmental items. Perhaps the chief reason for this was that progress in weight was apparent from day to day, whereas days and frequently weeks passed without the appearance of a new developmental item on the check list. The mothers were told that they should check a developmental item the first time it was noticed and for about two weeks following until they were sure the reaction was established. Some mothers followed these instructions closely and checked an item almost daily for two weeks. Some checked these items only once a week and as a rule checked the item for three or four successive weeks. Still others checked an item only at its first appearance, and several checked every reaction they noticed every day throughout the entire period. This latter method is undoubtedly the most reliable, but the examiners felt that it was too much to ask of busy mothers.

In dealing with the mothers' records it was decided that a reaction should be considered established if it had been checked eight times within two successive weeks or if it had been checked each week for three successive weeks. The age in weeks at the beginning of the consistent checking of the item was considered as the age at which the reaction was established. The data from the mothers' records leave much to be desired in the way of objectivity both because of the different methods of checking and because of the mothers' different interpretations of the items. If a mother expressed doubt as to the meaning of an item the examiners gave her their interpretation of it. In general the items were simply stated, and the best records came from mothers who took the items literally and naïvely checked them according to what each saw her baby do without any qualms as to her own ability to observe and interpret her baby's behavior.

Incidental Items

As has been explained in the previous chapter, the observers attempted to record not only the baby's reaction to each test situation but also all his other reactions during the examination. Each incidental item was copied from the original record on a card, and the items were classified into several categories. One of the largest categories was gross bodily movement. These cards contained records of all the rolling, creeping, standing, climbing reactions observed during the anthropometric and physical examinations during which no motor tests were given, and they also recorded all the motor items observed during the psychological examinations other than those in response to the motor tests. These incidental items contained not only additional information on creeping, sitting, and walking, but they were also the source of most of the data on motor play. Play information was recorded not only for the limited period of the test but for every moment the child was under observation. It included such items as: "runs to door to greet us"; "lifts head and smiles when B goes to crib"; "was bouncing in baby swing when we arrived"; "arches self on B's hands like athletic dancer, supported only at abdomen"; "follows us to door on kiddy-car when we leave"; and "stands at window waving bye-bye to us." Other items on motor play were obtained from the mothers' records. Items other than those in the check list were copied and classified as incidental items.

Combining Data from the Three Sources

The evaluation and weighing of data from the three sources presented some difficulties. Obviously the most objective data were obtained from the motor tests. But occasionally babies who were able to do the tests for some unknown reason refused to perform at their best in the test situation. All possible reactions to each test were recorded together with the ages at which each baby did them. To these were added the same reactions that occurred as incidental items. For example, one baby who did not creep at the motor test at 31 weeks, crept in the test given at 33 weeks. It was recorded at 32 weeks as an incidental item that he "rolled over on bed and crept away while B was measuring him." Hence, creeping was recorded first for him at 32 weeks. If the age given by the mother for a motor function differed greatly from the one recorded by the examiners, it was thought that her interpretation of the item was different from theirs, and her record was disregarded. If the age she gave coincided with that of the examiners, there was no question about the matter. When a long gap in the psychological examinations occurred — because of illness of the baby, members of his family, or the examiners, or because of the family's temporary absence from the city — and the observers noted at the next examination a new reaction that the mother had recorded as having been established two or three weeks earlier, her record was taken as the true date.

Some criticism may be raised with these methods of combining the data. The data would have been much easier to handle if only those reactions that occurred at the test had been studied. It was felt, however, that the important fact was that the baby rolled over, crept, or climbed by holding to furniture, rather than that he rolled, crept, or climbed at the test situation. Since the object of this study of motor development was to study the child's true motor ability rather than his artificially elicited performance, it was thought best to include all available data. This method of combining data was far from perfect, but it was the most satisfactory method that could be devised.

CHAPTER III

PROGRESS TOWARD CREEPING

The fact that the observers were unable to devise a simple and practical way of measuring progress toward creeping and as a result had to content themselves with brief descriptive accounts has already been dwelt upon. The next difficulty to be met was that of deciding if a given reaction represented a step in the creeping sequence or if it belonged more properly to the progress in sitting or walking. It goes without saying that motor development was rather more general than specific and that any new phase of motor skill probably contributed alike to progress in creeping, sitting, standing, and walking. Nevertheless, to simplify the analysis of motor development it was necessary to consider the three or four aspects of development separately. The reactions chosen as contributing most toward progress in creeping were those that occurred in the tests with the baby lying on his stomach and those that involved turning and rolling responses when he was lying on his back. Similar reactions gleaned from incidental items and mothers' records were also included in the data on creeping.

All of the babies went through almost the same series of reactions in approximately the same order. Their earliest reaction when they were in a prone position was turning the head to free the nose for breathing. Later they went through stages of lifting the head so that the chin was free, raising the chest, making swimming movements with the arms and legs, rolling, rocking, or pivoting on the stomach so that some progress was made, scooting or sliding backward, and creeping forward on hands and knees. The ages at which the babies representing the median and the first and third quartiles reached each stage are given in Table I.

TABLE I

THE MEDIAN AND QUARTILE AGES FOR THE BEGINNING OF EACH STAGE OF THE CREEPING SEQUENCE

Description of Stage	No. of Cases	Age in Weeks		
		Q_1	Median	Q_3
Chin up	22	2.0	3.0	7.0
Chest up	22	5.0	9.0	10.0
Knee push or swim	22	22.0	25.0	27.0
Rolling	19	25.0	29.0	32.0
Rock or pivot; some progress	17	32.5	37.0	41.0
Scoot backward	16	34.0	39.5	45.5
Creep	22	41.0	44.5	45.0

Motor Development Considered as a Direct Function of Age

For the sake of graphic representation all motor development was considered as a direct function of age. This assumption may not be true, to be sure, but age from birth was the only scale available. Objections to it may be raised on the ground that the ages of babies as reckoned from time of conception varies greatly at birth and that age from conception would be the better age measure. Without elaborate tests, however, it is impossible to determine the amount of prematurity or postmaturity of an infant at birth, and estimated age from conception would have been less objective than calculated age from birth. For lack of any better measure of maturity age from birth was used throughout the study.

In graphic representation of all facts for which no other scale is available the age scale is used for both axes as in Figure 1. Age in weeks is plotted along the axis of abscissas. The units along the axis of ordinates are made equal in size to the week unit of the abscissas. The heavier lines drawn at irregular intervals along this scale represent stages of progress in motor skills, and the ordinate height of each line represents the median age of the babies at reaching each level of performance. The spread of the middle 50 per cent of the group in age of attaining each stage in creeping is depicted by the bars in Figure 1. The width of the bar indicates the distance between the first and third quartiles, its height indicates the function developed, and the point at which the 45-degree angle line cuts the top of the bar marks the median. The fact that bars are used indicates that the observations were recorded in discontinuous steps rather than on a continuous scale.

The Creeping Sequence in Detail

Body postures and motor performance during hospital period. — The commonest posture of the newborn baby when sleeping on his back was with knees somewhat flexed, arms flexed at the elbow, upper arm close to the sides, palms facing outward, fists closed, and hands lying at the shoulder level. When the baby was awake he turned his head freely from right to left and did much random kicking and squirming, particularly if he were crying. A few babies turned completely from the back to the side; such reactions were observed in six babies between the ages of 1 and 11 days, and in one baby it was observed twice during the hospital period. Still another made a turn at 3 weeks. Five babies made a turn from side to back or stomach in the early weeks, but this reaction was probably passive, a result of losing balance when lying on the side and hence of toppling over.

FIGURE 1

PROGRESS TOWARD CREEPING

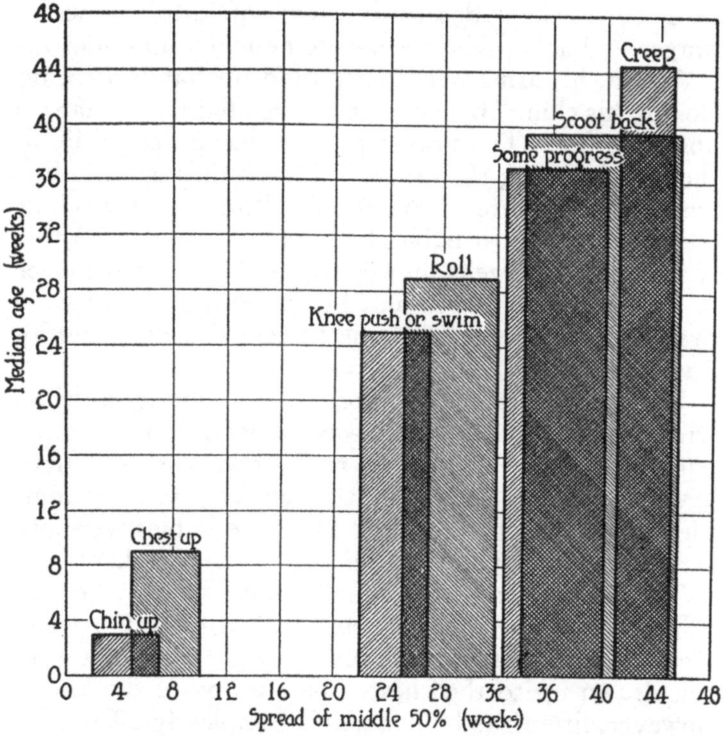

The units on both the horizontal and vertical axes represent age in weeks. The height of a bar is determined by the median age at which the stage it represents was developed. The width of a bar indicates the spread of the middle 50 per cent of the babies at the age of development represented. The heights of the bars thus give some idea of the relative difficulty of each stage of development, and the widths depict variability in the age of development of each stage.

Characteristically the newborn baby curled up in a posture similar to that of the fetus before birth when he was placed on his stomach. Examiner B gave this posture the excellent descriptive term of "Mohammedan prayer." The baby's knees were hunched up under his abdomen, his arms were flexed, and his hands were up close to his chin. His face was turned slightly so that his nose was free. The prayer posture was observed in all the babies during the first few days, and it is well illustrated in a picture of Winifred at the age of 7 weeks (see Plate 1). Most babies had gradually outgrown this stage by 3 or 4 weeks, but it persisted somewhat longer in two babies, Winifred and Edith, both of whom were premature, the former by 6 or 7 weeks and the latter by 2 weeks.

Rolling from the prayer position was simple; a thrust with one foot was all that was necessary to upset the equilibrium, and the infant rolled to his back. Fred, aged 8 days, was caught by the camera just as he completed such a roll (see Plate 1). Five babies were observed to roll in this way before the 12th week.

The prayer position gradually gave way as the legs relaxed from their flexed neonatal posture. For some time the knees remained flexed at a right angle but were not drawn up to the chest. The flexing of the knees, however, lifted the baby's pelvis completely off the table. This posture was called "rooting" since the baby often squirmed about and nuzzled the blanket with his head. Caroline, aged 2 days, went so far as to push with her toes, thus lifting her trunk completely off the table, and at 6 days she squirmed enough to progress a few inches along the table.

The kicking of very young babies was fairly strong. At 2 days Don kicked the examiner soundly, and at 5

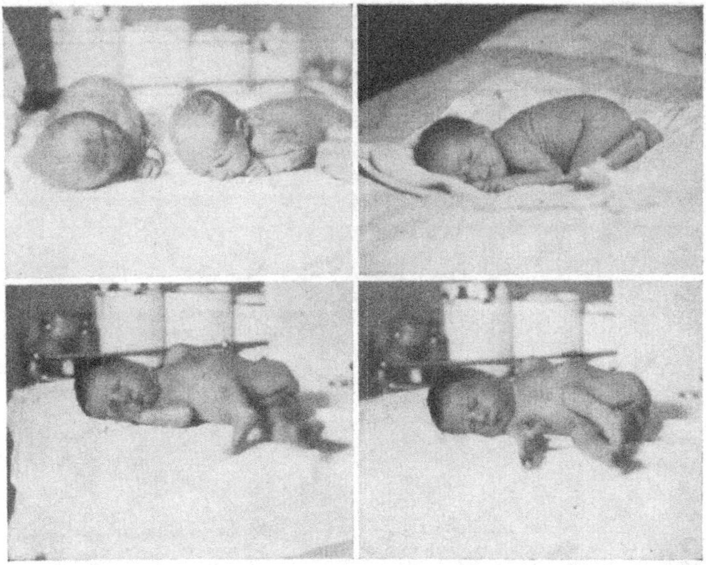

PLATE 1. — ACTIVITIES OF NEWBORNS

Upper left. — Peter and Patty at 4 days. Note their flexed arms and hunched backs. *Upper right.* — Mohammedan prayer: Winifred at 7 weeks. *Lower left.* — Fred executes a roll from abdomen to side at 8 days. Note the left toes pushing and right hand rubbing his nose. *Lower right.* — As he completes the roll he draws up his left foot, stretches his right arm, and fans out the fingers.

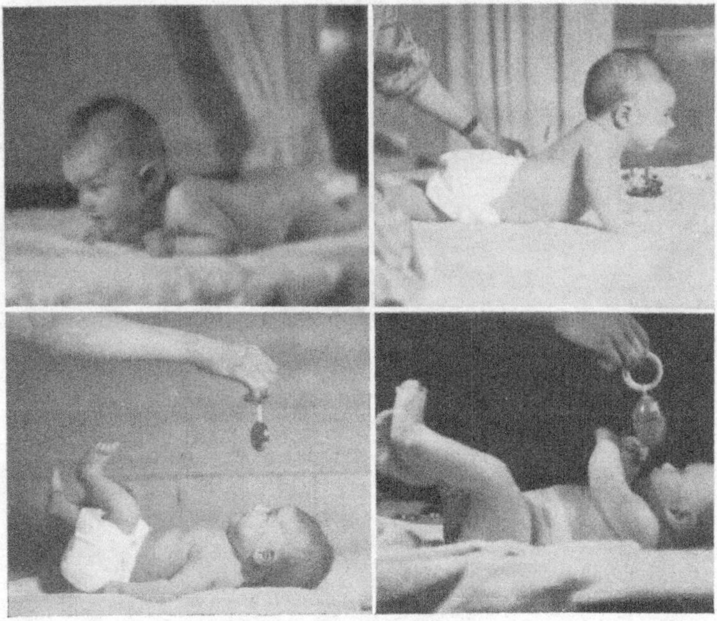

Plate 2. — Early Lying Postures

Upper left. — Chin up: Judy at 14 weeks. *Upper right.* — Chest up: Don at 9 weeks. *Lower left.* — Interested watching: Doris at 9 weeks. *Lower right.* — Hands and feet both work: Irene May at 14 weeks.

days he almost turned over by kicking. Fred was observed to kick his feet alternately and rhythmically at the age of 10 days. Virginia Ruth at 3 weeks kicked so hard against the observer's abdomen that she pushed the light nursery table on which she was lying a few inches in the opposite direction.

These early motor reactions were not indicative of precocity in motor development. In fact some of the babies who did seemingly remarkable rolling and lifting accomplished these feats in spite of their weakness and prematurity, or perhaps because of it. Although all babies kicked vigorously, it was generally the smaller ones who turned and rolled.

Lifting the head: chin up, chest up. — The first marked advance came when the baby lifted his head from the table far enough to free his chin. (See Plate 2.) Most babies lifted the head momentarily during the 1st or 2nd week. Three weeks was the median age at which the head-lifting reaction was established; by 7 weeks three-fourths of the babies had achieved this skill. The chest-lifting reaction had two variations, one in which the chest was lifted, the weight being supported by the elbows and forearm, and a second in which the baby supported himself with his hands (Plate 2, upper right). The chest-lifting reaction was considered established if the baby persisted in it for one minute. Half of the babies reached this level of proficiency at or before 9 weeks. These two items chin- and chest-lifting are included in the Gesell 4-month test, the first getting a rating of C and the second a rating of B. Observations on this group would indicate that the chin-up if not the chest-up reaction is too elementary for a diagnostic item at 4 months. For many weeks the baby did not advance beyond this point, except that he supported himself with his hands for longer periods and sometimes waved his feet in the air or dug his toes into the blanket or rug and gave a little push.

Drawing up the knees: swimming. — The baby's next effort consisted in drawing up the legs frog-like and in kicking them out suddenly as if swimming. Frequently there was great straining and reaching with the arms, particularly if the baby were headed toward an attractive toy. If progress were made at all by this method, it was usually in the backward direction. The abdomen was not lifted off the floor, and the hands and feet often worked at cross purposes. Frequently babies who were thus struggling for the bell pulled a corner of the creeping blanket and thus brought the toy within reach. Reactions falling in this category were established at a median age of 25 weeks.

Rolling. — In general the complete roll did not appear before the baby was 6 months old. An easy roll from the back was often achieved by the baby's flexing his hips and stretching out his legs at right angles to the trunk. The roll that was done by simply twisting the pelvis was seldom noticed in babies of this age. The median baby rolled from back to stomach at the age of 29 weeks.

Hitching on the back. — An interesting reaction that occurred in too few babies to be considered an important step toward locomotion was that of hitching on the back. At the age of 20 weeks Patricia hitched the length of the dining-room table and was caught only on the brink of a fall. Her method, although effective and apparently easy for her, would have meant torture to an adult. She flexed her knees and set her feet flat on the floor, then drew back her head and arched her neck and back so that she was propped on the crown of her head and the soles of her feet. She then inched along by repeatedly lifting her feet and setting them down each time closer to her trunk. Thus she plowed along on her head with considerable speed and steered a fairly straight course. Another baby made progress on his back by drawing his feet up in the same way and lifting his buttocks off the floor. He thus hitched from side to side, but his shoulders remained in place as a pivot. Still others made a heel-to-head arch according to reports of the mothers, but none traveled so skillfully as did Patricia.

Some progress in a prone position. — Most of the babies devised some way of making progress before they were actually able to creep. As long as the abdomen and pelvis weighted them down they could make little headway. Many of them, however, rocked back and forth on their stomachs. Frequently the stomach served as a pivot; the baby supported himself with his hands, lifted his legs from the floor, and by pushing and reaching sometimes made a right-angle turn. At 37 weeks the median baby was covering some distance forward, backward, or sidewise, when he was put on the floor for crawling.

"*Suspension-bridge*" *reaction.* — A reaction similar to that of lifting on the heels and head when on the back was the "suspension-bridge" reaction. From a position on his stomach the baby shifted his weight to hands and toes and suspended his body in mid-air for a moment. An excellent movie of this reaction was obtained on Winifred. Eight babies in all were caught doing a suspension-bridge stunt either by the observers or by their mothers. It is possible that the reaction occurred in more of the babies but that it was overlooked by the mothers because it had not been anticipated when the items for the mothers' record blanks were compiled. The median age at which the babies exhibited the suspension bridge was 38 weeks. Most of these babies crept about two weeks after they performed this stunt.

Scooting backwards. — The final step before creeping was scooting backwards. This reaction usually occurred inadvertently when the baby was attempting to get up on his hands and knees to creep or to push to a sitting posture. The baby first propped himself on his hands and walked his hands backward toward his knees, thus lifting his pelvis from the floor. Usually, however, before he got to the creeping or sitting position he had scooted backward some distance on the floor. The median age for scooting backwards was 39.5 weeks. Some babies became very proficient at this crawfish method of locomotion. The mother of Irene May reported that the little girl usually made no effort to creep when she was on the floor, but if she saw a toy that she wanted she promptly faced about and backed up to it.

Creeping and hitching. — Since each baby had slightly different ways of creeping, the term "creeping" is used here to mean any type of locomotion whereby the baby covered the ground and made real progress about the house. One baby, Nathaniel, rolled from room to room, cleverly turning corners, escaping furniture, and piloting himself through narrow doorways. Harvey made his first real progress by crawling or swimming across the floor. He folded his arms in front of him and, propping himself on his forearms, used them as levers or paddles to pull himself forward. Four babies, Doris, Larry, Matthew, and Sibyl hitched in the sitting posture before they crept on hands and knees. Matthew's method was most ingenious. He sat with his right leg doubled under him, his left knee flexed, and his left foot flat on the floor.

His hands were on the floor with fingers turned in, and he walked forward stepping first with his hands and then with his left foot. Incidentally he wore off all the skin on his right leg, which bore the brunt of whatever rough going was in his path.

In general the hitching, rolling, and swimming types of locomotion seemed to be more primitive than creeping on hands and knees. Although they were often quite as effective methods of covering the ground, they were usually abandoned for regular creeping after a few weeks. The median age for creeping was 44.5 weeks.

Consistency of the Sequence

One may question how closely each baby followed the sequence of steps in the creeping progress and whether each step and its position in the sequence was an essential part of a creeping pattern that was fixed and inflexible. The number of cases listed for each stage appear in Table I. No stage was listed as a characteristic part of the progress unless it was observed in sixteen of the twenty-two babies. From Figure 1 it will be seen that there is some overlapping of the middle 50 per cent of the group between the stages of swimming and rolling and between the stages of making some progress, scooting backward, and creeping. There was, however, no exception to the rule that chin-lifting preceded chest-lifting and that chest-lifting preceded knee push or swim. With fourteen of nineteen babies the swimming stage preceded that of rolling, and with one baby the two stages were observed simultaneously. For fifteen babies rolling preceded the stage of making some progress; for only two babies was the order reversed. In every case some progress preceded the stage called scooting backward, although backward progress was sometimes achieved by sliding during the swimming or pivoting stage. Scooting backward was confined to progress on the hands and knees. Finally, scooting backward preceded creeping in all cases but two, and in those the two performances appeared at the same age.

The only argument for saying that each stage is an essential one in the creeping process is that with rare exceptions each baby goes through all of them, and the argument for calling the sequence of stages a pattern is that each baby progresses through the stages in the same order regardless of the speed at which he is developing. To be sure, the stages are rather widely spaced, a fact that gives little chance for reversals in the order. Very probably there are other stages of importance that the methods of these tests did not elicit. But on the whole it seems safe to conclude that development toward creeping proceeds in an orderly and fairly fixed way for all babies.

CHAPTER IV

ASSUMING AN UPRIGHT POSTURE

Stages in Progress toward Standing Erect

Progress in assuming an upright posture was as unmeasurable as was progress in creeping. It could be observed only in spurts and stages and could be recorded only in descriptive terms. In deciding which reactions belonged to the sequence of standing erect, subjective judgment again had to be relied upon. All reactions to the lying-on-the-back test except that of rolling were put into this sequence. These reactions consisted in tensing the muscles for lifting and in lifting the head from the floor. All reactions to the sitting and standing tests were placed in this sequence. The various stages of the sequence in order of their appearance were:

1. Tensing the muscles for being lifted
2. Sitting on the examiner's lap with a standard amount of support
3. Lifting the head from the floor spontaneously
4. Sitting alone momentarily
5. Standing with support at the armpits
6. Sitting alone for one minute
7. Standing by holding to furniture
8. Sitting down from standing by furniture
9. Pulling self to standing position by means of furniture
10. Standing alone

Pushing self to sitting posture properly belongs in this sequence but the data on this point were too incomplete to include it. Table II gives the median and quartile ages for each stage in the sequence; Figure 2 presents the data graphically on a scale similar to that used in Figure 1.

Tensing for being lifted.—Both the mothers and the observers tested and recorded this stage by noting whether the baby made a preliminary shoulder adjustment when the hands were slipped under his back. In general the mothers reported this act as established at an earlier age

TABLE II

THE MEDIAN AND QUARTILE AGES FOR THE BEGINNING OF EACH STAGE TOWARD ASSUMING ERECT POSTURE

Description of Stage	No. of Cases	Age in Weeks		
		Q_1	Median	Q_3
Tense for lifting..........	19	14.0	15.0	18.0
Sit on lap...............	22	15.0	18.5	19.5
Sit alone momentarily.....	22	20.5	25.0	26.0
Sit alone 1 minute........	20	27.0	31.0	34.0
Stand holding to furniture.	22	41.0	42.0	45.0
Pull to stand by furniture..	17	42.0	47.0	49.5
Stand alone.............	21	56.0	62.0	66.0

than did the observers. Since some mothers omitted this item altogether and since each mother probably interpreted the item differently, only the records of the observers were considered. According to their observation adjustment was made by the median baby at 15 weeks.

Sitting on the lap.—Sitting on the lap was estimated on a somewhat finer scale than were the other reactions. In order to make it comparable with other items a special criterion for sitting on the lap was adopted, namely, that the baby sit on the examiner's lap throughout a ten-minute test with support at the lower ribs and with complete head control. The babies met this criterion at a median age of 18.5 weeks. Sitting propped up with pillows was one of the items noted by the mothers, and according to their reports the median age for establish-

FIGURE 2

ASSUMING AN UPRIGHT POSTURE

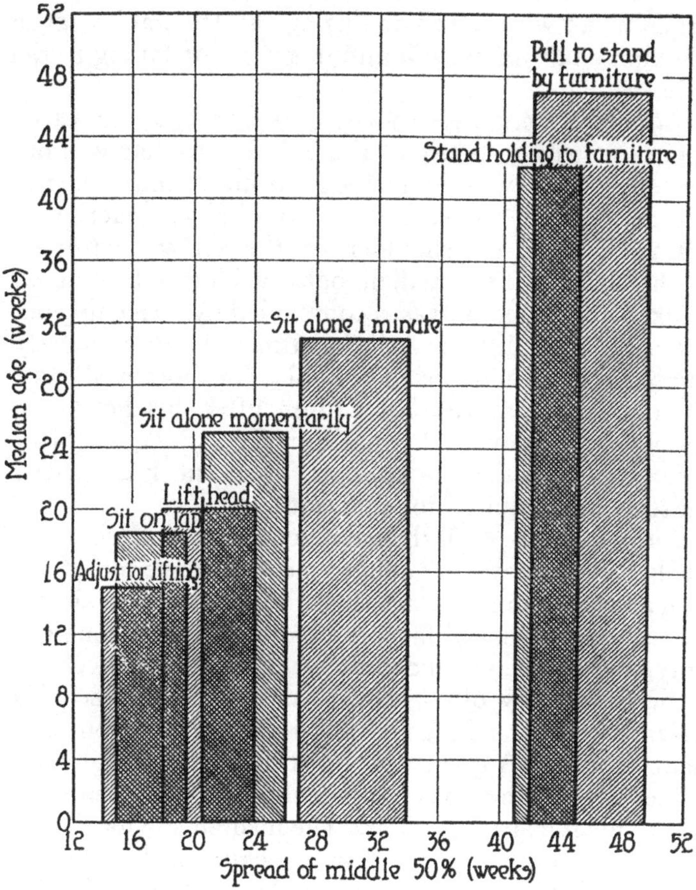

ing this skill was 15 weeks. Sitting in a high chair for periods of fifteen to thirty minutes was established shortly before 6 months. No test was made for this particular function, but the high chair was used for choice tests that began at 25 weeks, and at this age all the babies sat in the high chair for several minutes without falling to the side.

Lifting the head. — Another reaction that appeared spontaneously in many of the babies but that was observed in too few to be included as an essential part of the developmental pattern was the baby's reaction of lifting the head and shoulders off the pillow when lying on his back. The median baby achieved this at 20 weeks. Sometimes it was accompanied by stretching out the arms to be lifted. At other times the baby merely raised his head and looked around. The mother of Martin reported that the baby often lifted his head and shoulders and lay in this position for as long as thirty seconds. Considerable strength of the neck and back muscles was required for this feat.

Sitting alone. — All the babies could sit alone momentarily before they were able to meet the criterion of sitting a whole minute. Once this criterion was met, sitting was an accomplished fact; the baby could sit alone not only one minute but indefinitely. In the early weeks of sitting the baby often leaned far forward to keep his balance. At first he could not raise himself from this bent posture. A great deal of skill at sitting had been achieved when he was able to bend and straighten himself to his full sitting height. The median age for sitting alone one minute was 31 weeks. Rocking back and forth in the sitting posture was a playful stunt indulged in by many babies shortly after they had begun to sit alone well. Various stages of sitting are illustrated in Plates 3 and 4.

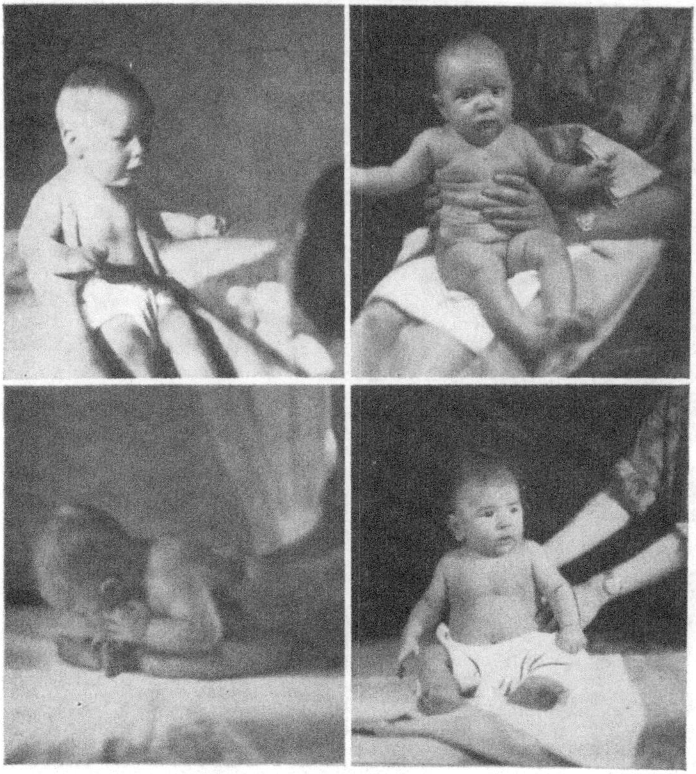

PLATE 3. — SITTING WITH SUPPORT

Upper left. — Tense for being lifted: David at 11 weeks. *Upper right.* — Support at the midribs: Irene May at 14 weeks. *Lower left.* — Getting acquainted with toes: Judy at 14 weeks. *Lower right.* — Sitting almost unsupported: Rex at 12 weeks.

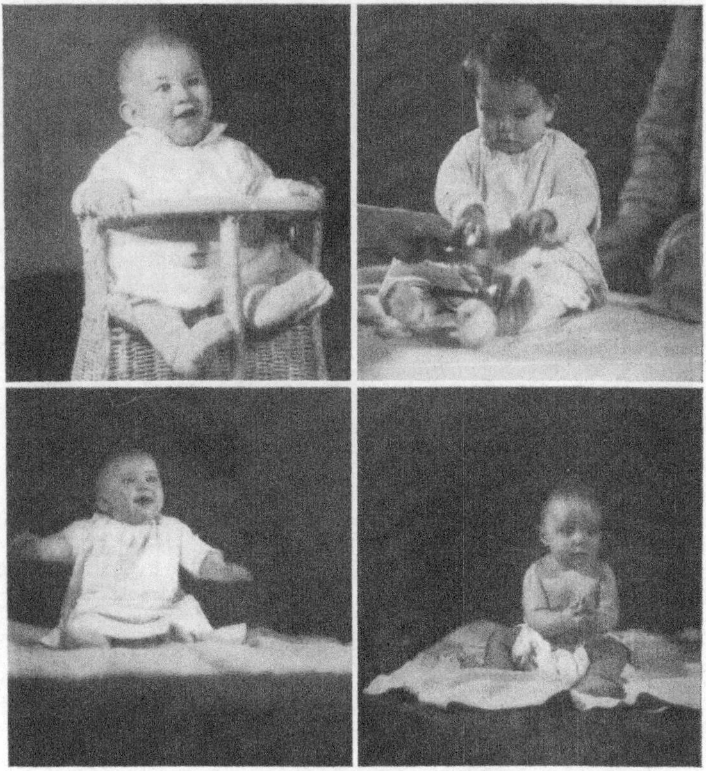

PLATE 4. — SITTING ALONE

Upper left. — Graduated to high chair: Larry at 31 weeks. *Upper right.* — A little unsteady: Edith Ann at 34 weeks. *Lower left.* — All alone: Carol at 34 weeks. *Lower right.* — Legs outstretched for balancing: Irene May at 36 weeks.

Standing by furniture; lowering to sit and raising to stand. — Standing by furniture was considerably easier than pulling to the standing position. The median baby met the one-minute criterion for standing by furniture at 42 weeks; as he perfected the skill he leaned less and less heavily on the chair and frequently let go completely for the twinkling of an eye. Shortly after the babies became proficient at standing several were observed to lower themselves slowly and carefully to the sitting posture, but there are too few records of this feat to include it in the developmental scheme. In general it came about two weeks later than the standing stage. When the babies discovered that they could sit down again after they had obtained the toy it was usually impossible to get them to stand for an entire minute. In pulling to the standing posture the baby met with many vicissitudes. Often his legs slid completely under the chair. If he got up to his knees he was sometimes able to reach the bell without getting to his feet. Pulling to a standing position was established for the median baby at 47 weeks.

Standing alone. — Standing alone was not observed in most babies until they were able to walk alone.

Pattern in the Development of Erect Posture

Reactions leading to an upright posture begin at the head and proceed down the neck and trunk to the legs. At birth the baby has no control over his head and neck muscles; when he is held upright he cuddles on the nurse's bosom and rests his head on her shoulder. If he is held out from the nurse's body, he has to be given support at the head and neck. In a short time he achieves control over the head and neck muscles, and the nurse's hands need only to be placed at the nape of the neck, later at the shoulder blades, still later in the thoracic and lumbar regions, and finally under his buttocks only. The varying degrees of support necessary to keep the baby sitting upright on the lap also illustrate the principle that the baby begins assuming an erect posture at the head and gradually works downward. Lifting the head and shoulders indicates that these parts have come under control. It is interesting to note that about five-months arm control is manifested by the ability to reach and grasp objects. In general, skill with the arm is achieved at about the age the baby meets the criterion for sitting on the lap, or in other words when postural control has progressed as far as the mid-trunk region.

In order for the baby to sit alone the entire trunk must be under control. With the baby who is almost, but not quite, able to sit alone it is the lower part of the trunk that gives way and not the upper. Leaning forward, which is characteristic of this period, is a way of getting more support for the lower trunk. The legs are not straightened for standing until the trunk is well under control.

The sequence of steps toward upright posture seems to follow the same law as that for anatomical growth. The law that growth begins cephelad and proceeds caudad has long been established. The development of function, especially as it is illustrated by upright posture, appears to proceed in the same way. Not only does development of uprightness follow a pattern, but the pattern takes on meaning in the light of anatomical growth.

CHAPTER V

DEVELOPMENT OF WALKING

Walking is certainly the most spectacular and probably the most important single phase of motor development. From time immemorial parents have looked upon baby's first step as a milestone long to be remembered. Psychologists likewise have recognized the importance of this function. The age of walking is usually listed as a normative item in tests for young children, but in spite of its obvious importance only a few studies of walking development have been made, and these, for the most part, have been based on a few observations of less than a dozen children.

Burnside's study of locomotion (8), which appeared shortly before this work was started, was suggestive as to method, and it was with the hope of verifying her results on a larger scale that the walking records were begun. Thanks to a method of recording footprints, differing only slightly from that of Burnside, the observers were able to collect a large mass of objective data on walking. Hence this phase of motor development will be considered in greater detail than progress toward creeping and sitting.

The object of this study is to analyze the course of the walking process from 4 months to 2 years in order to: (1) trace the stages of development in walking; (2) discover factors or elements that contribute to progress in acquisition of walking skill, such as speed of walking, length of step, width of step, angle of step, in-toeing and out-toeing; (3) study individual differences in walking;

(4) discuss the significance of the pattern of walking development.

Method of Studying Walking

Analysis can be made only after systematic observation of a group of babies from the time they first pat their feet and bounce when they are held erect upon a flat surface up to the time they run about the house, the complete masters of their legs.

Technique of Record-Taking[1]

Interval of testing. — The observations on walking were made at regular weekly or biweekly intervals on all the babies in the infant-study group. During the first year the physical examinations and the measurements made a long and difficult siege for the baby, and since these came only once in four weeks it was thought unnecessary to prolong them by the walking test. Thus records were obtained for three out of every four weeks during the first year. During the second year the walking test was taken at the end of each biweekly examination regardless of its type. The babies were on the average 17 weeks (4 months) old when the first record was taken. Complete records were obtained on twenty babies from 17 to 78 weeks (18 months) and on seventeen babies up to 104 weeks (2 years). Occasional illnesses on the part of the baby made gaps in his record, and several long omissions in the records during the second year were caused by the babies' leaving town for the summer vacation. During the second year two babies showed fear or abandoned themselves to fits of temper whenever

[1] The author is indebted to Mr. Donovan Lawrence, technician of the Institute of Child Welfare, for devising this method for taking graphic records of walking.

they saw the paper, and the walking test had to be discontinued for a few weeks until they overcame their dislike for it. Throughout the entire two-year period 743 graphic records were collected.

Graphic record of footprints. — A graphic record of the baby's walking was obtained at each test by the following simple method: a strip of unglazed white wrapping paper twelve inches wide was stretched out the length of the living-room floor. The soles of the baby's feet were lightly greased with olive oil and he walked along the paper path. At the end of the day's examinations these oil print records were taken to the laboratory and brushed over with a powder of lamp black, graphite, and powdered acacia. The black powder adhered to the oil and made the footprints stand out clearly.

Handling the baby. — Up to the time they walked alone the babies had to be supported for the walking test. From the beginning of the tests to 32 weeks the examiner gave the baby support by placing her hands just under his armpits and holding him thus with his feet touching the paper. Since the baby needed less support after 32 weeks to keep himself in an upright position, the examiner held him by grasping his hands at the wrists and extending her fingers along his arms to give him support until he could walk alone. After the baby walked alone he sometimes had to be led by one hand or gently steered by a hand at his back to keep him on the paper. Frequently he was given the oil bottle, a favorite toy with all the babies, and told to take it to Examiner S, who stood at the end of the path. Many babies grasped the idea of walking on the paper and required no assistance.

One examiner held a stop watch and kept time at the walking test. During the first year the baby was allowed to walk for one minute, but at the beginning of the second year the babies were traveling such long distances in one minute that the most spacious living rooms and halls were not long enough for their walking paths. Consequently the walking path was made a convenient length of about three meters, long enough to get at least ten steps from the baby. The baby was lifted off the path after five, ten, or fifteen seconds, according to his walking speed. In subsequent computations walking distance and number of steps were prorated on the basis of one minute. The examiner recorded on the walking paper the baby's name and age, the date, the length of time allowed for the record, and significant notes on the baby's skill and attitude at the walking test.

Measuring the Records

In the early weeks many babies danced and patted with only their toes touching the paper; no heel marks were made. Therefore it was necessary to use toe prints rather than heel prints as a point of reference in the measurement of the early records, and since this method was used at the start it was adhered to throughout. All the distances were measured with the metric scale. The measurements were made as shown in Figure 3.

Enumeration of prints. — All footprints were counted and labeled right or left, and records were made of: (1) total footprints made with right, with left, and with both feet; (2) total prints of right, left, and both feet in which the full foot was visible; (3) total prints of right, left, and both feet in which the toes only were visible; (4) total prints of right, left, and both feet in which the sides of the foot only were visible.

Total distance traversed. — The distance in centimeters was measured between a line drawn perpendicular to the walking path at the tip of the first visible toe print

FIGURE 3

DIAGRAM SHOWING THE METHOD OF MEASURING FOOTPRINTS

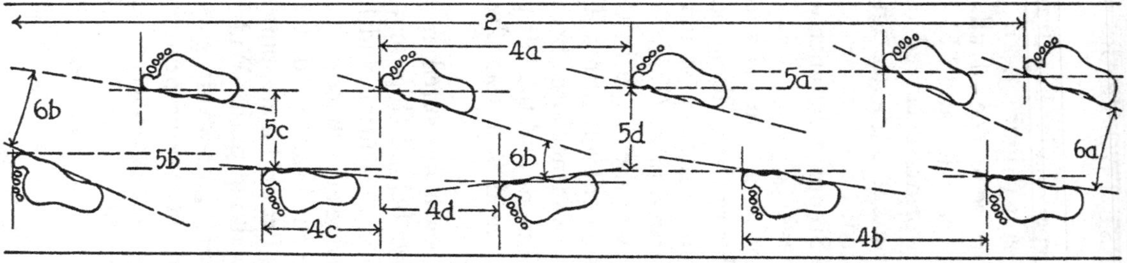

2 total distance traversed
4a right-right step length
4b left-left step length
4c right-left step length
4d left-right step length

5a right-right step width
5b left-left step width
5c right-left step width
5d left-right step width
6a standing angle

6b stepping angle

and a corresponding perpendicular line drawn at the tip of the last visible toe print (Figure 3, 2).

Print sequence. — The sequence of all visible footprints was recorded as "r," "l," and "b" according to the order in which the prints occurred on the paper. The total number of prints in sequence agreed with the number of prints counted.

Stepping distance. — Stepping distance was measured in the following four ways:

1. Right-right distance was the distance between a line drawn perpendicular to the walking path at the tip of the first right-toe print and a line similarly drawn at the tip of the next right-toe print (Figure 3, 4a).

2. Left-left distance was measured in the same way from toe to toe of subsequent left prints (Figure 3, 4b).

3. Right-left distance was measured between the perpendiculars of the right print and the left print just following it. The foot named first was always the foot behind (Figure 3, 4c).

4. Left-right distance was measured in the same way with the left foot always behind (Figure 3, 4d).

Stepping width. — For measuring widths lines were drawn along the inner edge of each footprint so that they touched the margins of the big-toe prints and were perpendicular to the lines drawn for stepping distance and hence parallel to the walking path. Widths were then measured in the following four ways:

1. Right-right width was the perpendicular distance between the width lines for two succeeding right footprints. This distance was labeled "in" if the second print came in toward the body and "out" if the second print was farther out toward the edge of the path than that of the first foot (Figure 3, 5a).

2. Left-left width was a similar measurement for succeeding left footprints.

3. Right-left width was measured between the width lines for a right and a succeeding left foot. This distance was labeled "minus" if the feet were crossed, the right print appearing on the left side of the left foot. "Minus" distances occurred rather frequently in the early stages of walking.

4. Left-right distances were similar measures taken with the left foot behind.

Angles. — For measuring angles a line was drawn along the inner margin of each footprint so that it touched the margin of the big toe and the inner edge of the heel print. The line was extended till it intersected the angle line for the foot preceding and the foot following the one in question. The size of each angle was measured in degrees and labeled "plus" if the prints were out-toeing and "minus" if they were pigeon-toeing. Positive angles of less than 12 degrees were considered straight and were not measured, but all negative angles were measured regardless of size:

1. The standing angle was measured between the first visible right and left prints (Figure 3, 6a).

2. Stepping angles were measured for each succeeding right-left and left-right step (Figure 3, 6b).

Notes. — All notes recorded on the graphic print record were copied verbatim on the sheet containing the measurements.

Pats. — Frequently the baby stood on one foot and patted the other several times before he made a real step. The number of prints appearing in each siege of patting were counted as accurately as possible and included in the total print count and in the print sequence. The number of pats was also recorded separately, but there was no attempt to measure them.

Pigeon-toeing. — Each step, which of course included two succeeding footprints, was scrutinized to see whether it was pigeon-toeing, straight, or out-toeing, and the total number of each type was recorded.

Up to the end of the first year the entire record for each baby at each week was measured in this detailed way. After one year, however, the babies became less variable in their stepping as they gained proficiency at walking, and it seemed unnecessary to measure the entire record except for computing total distance traversed and total prints, both of which had to be prorated on the basis of sixty seconds. The first ten steps were used as sample measurements of steps and angles.

Summarizing the Records

Records for each baby. — A summary for each baby at each age was made by computing the median of the lengths, widths, and angles of steps. The medians for the right-right, the left-left, the right-left, the left-right, and the right-left and left-right combined, were computed for both length and width of steps. The median stepping angle was computed. All records for a single child were then summarized on one sheet.

Medians and averages for the group at each age level. — Summaries for the entire group of babies were made for each of fourteen items, one for total distance, one for total prints, five for stepping lengths, five for stepping widths, and two for stepping angles. These summaries were made week by week and the medians and averages were computed for each week on each item. When these summaries were plotted to show the course of development of the walking function, it was found that certain features that had stood out very clearly during repeated observations and had shown up when the prints were measured were obscured by the fact that age was the basis for computation. Although each baby went through about the same stages in acquiring proficiency at walking, each went through these stages at different ages and at different rates. The babies finally walked alone at ages varying from 50 to 76 weeks.

Recomputation of data with progress at walking constant. — Since the primary purpose of the study was to trace the course of development of the walking process rather than the relation of walking to age, it was necessary to equate the babies at a time when they were equal in walking skill rather than when they were equal in age. Consequently new summary sheets were made out for each of the fourteen items with the age at which each baby first walked alone as the point of reference. The records of the age of walking alone for all babies were aligned in a central column. The columns to the left of this were then headed "47, ... 3, 2, 1 weeks before walking alone," and those to the right were headed "2, 4, 6, ... 40 weeks after walking alone." Medians were then computed for each week. The median was used rather than the average in these computations because, considering the small number of cases and the large variability at each week, this statistic was more representative than an average. Because the age concept is a natural and convenient one, the material was again thrown onto the age basis by using 17 weeks, the median age at which the walking records were begun, and 64 weeks, the median age at which the babies walked alone, as points of reference.

RESULTS OF FOOTPRINT STUDY

Stages of Development in the Walking Process

When development was studied with the function of walking constant, four well-defined stages of progress were revealed as shown in Figure 4.

Early period of stepping. — The earliest stage was one in which the baby neither stiffened his knees nor supported his weight but instead danced and patted on the paper. Usually he made three or four swinging, lunging steps, thus progressing along the path a meter or more during the one-minute interval. All babies whose walking records were started before 20 weeks exhibited a stage of this sort. In general this stage began with the baby's first record at 17 weeks and lasted 11 weeks thereafter, or until 28 weeks. There was considerable variability in the age at which this period ended, the range being from 15 to 33 weeks.

Period of standing with support. — The second stage was one in which the baby stood with support, bearing most of his weight on his feet and tensing the muscles of his outstretched arms, which the examiner held, to keep from losing his balance. A few babies had reached this stage before their walking records were started and were standing well at the time of their first record at 21 weeks. Three babies did not show a period of this sort at all but from the first walking test on always made some progress. But eighteen babies did pass through a standing period that lasted for varying intervals of from 8 to 23 weeks. In median length this period was 14 weeks, extending from 28 to 42 weeks. This stage is an important step on the road to walking. The sooner it is reached the sooner the baby will walk alone, and the later it comes the more retarded he will be. A rank-order cor-

FIGURE 4

PROGRESS TOWARD WALKING

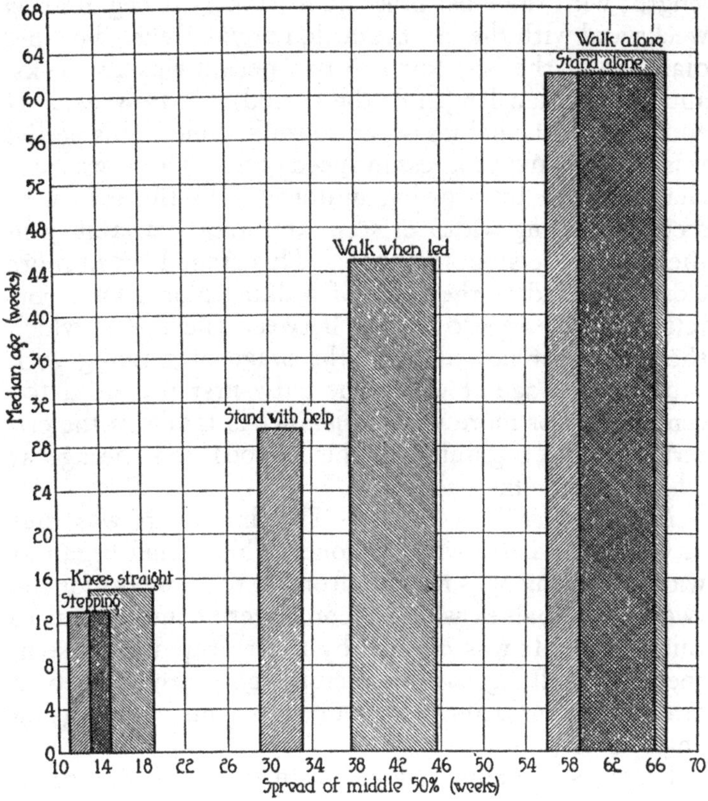

relation of $+.80 \pm .06$ exists between the age at which twenty babies reached the standing period and the age at which they walked alone.

Period of walking when led. — The third stage was one in which the babies walked when they were led by both hands. This period was of great variability in length; with the most precocious walkers it began at 23 weeks and with the most retarded at 72 weeks. The median age at the beginning of this period was 42 weeks, and the median length of the period was 22 weeks. It ended when the babies began to walk alone. This period was one of rapid progress in speed of walking; it was also characterized by growing uniformity in the length of step, increasing width of step, and great variability in the size of the stepping angle. This stage is even more closely related to the stage of walking alone, for a correlation of $+.91 \pm .03$ exists between the age at which the babies embarked upon the stage of walking with support (the age at which the baby first traversed 100 centimeters or more with assistance is taken as the criterion of the beginning of this period) and the age at which they walked alone.

Period of walking alone. — The final stage was that in which the baby walked alone. This period began at widely varying ages ranging from 50 to 76 weeks for the twenty-one babies whose records were complete up to this period. It was marked by a very rapid increase in speed of walking, by an increasing length of step, a gradually decreasing width of step, and a decreasing angle of step.

Progress in walking alone was manifested from 64 to 90 weeks. At the end of this 26-week period perfection in walking skill was reached, at least as far as it was indicated by the measurable items listed above. From 90

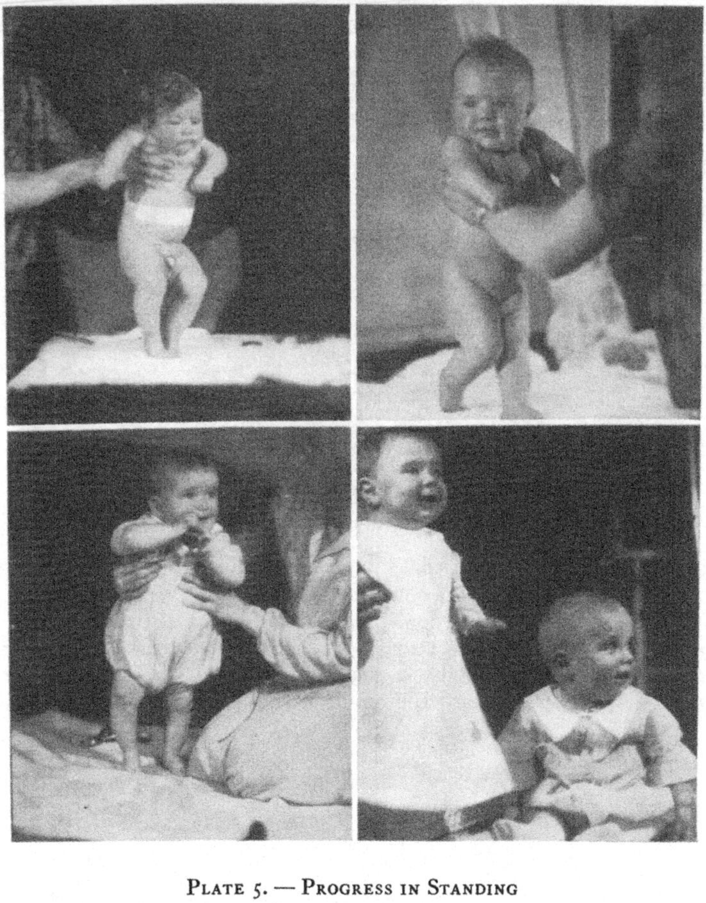

PLATE 5. — PROGRESS IN STANDING

Upper left. — Knees flexed, poised on toes: Torey at 16 weeks. *Upper right.* — Early stepping: Judy at 14 weeks. *Lower left.* — Standing with help: Max at 33 weeks. *Lower right.* — Patty and Peter at 33 weeks.

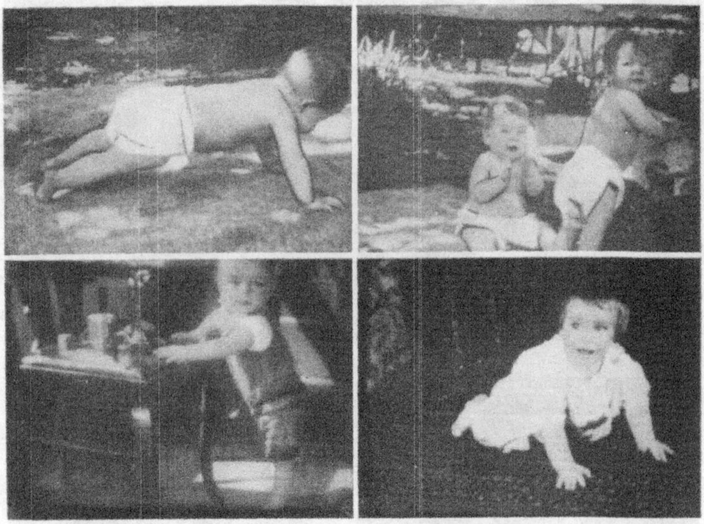

PLATE 6. — BABIES IN ACTION
(from a moving-picture film)

Upper left. — Suspension bridge: Winifred at 40 weeks. *Upper right.* — Winnie standing; Fred pat-a-caking at 40 weeks. *Lower left.* — Pulling to stand by a chair: Matthew at 51 weeks. *Lower right.* — Creeping toward the movie man: Nathaniel at 51 weeks.

to 104 weeks, the end of record-taking, the babies were on a plateau in walking skill so far as their records show. It is probable, however, that this lack of progress during the last three months of the second year is more apparent than it is real. The more plausible interpretation is that with increased skill in walking the joy in walking for its own sake decreased, and the test began to bore the baby. Some babies made clear their distaste for the test by refusing to walk on the paper. One or two babies ran the length of the paper path willingly enough, but they straddled the paper or walked at one side of it. Others occasionally introduced fancy steps into the prosaic old test by stamping or clumping along in a half-limping step. Several records were labeled as atypical and were not measured. Hence toward the end of the second year it was the baby's attitude toward the test and his mood or whim at the moment rather than his true skill at walking that was expressed in the walking record.

Development in Various Phases That Contribute to Skill in Walking

The development in each phase of the walking process can be explained more easily by reference to the charts.

Total distance traversed. — Before the data for total distance traversed were plotted the medians for each week were smoothed by using a five-point running average for the data collected at weekly intervals and a three-point running average for those collected at biweekly intervals. The progress in walking as measured by the distance traversed in a one-minute interval is depicted in Figure 5. In the early period of stepping about 60 centimeters in distance was covered at each weekly examination. The onset of the period of standing was

FIGURE 5

MEDIAN DISTANCE TRAVERSED IN A ONE-MINUTE INTERVAL OF WALKING

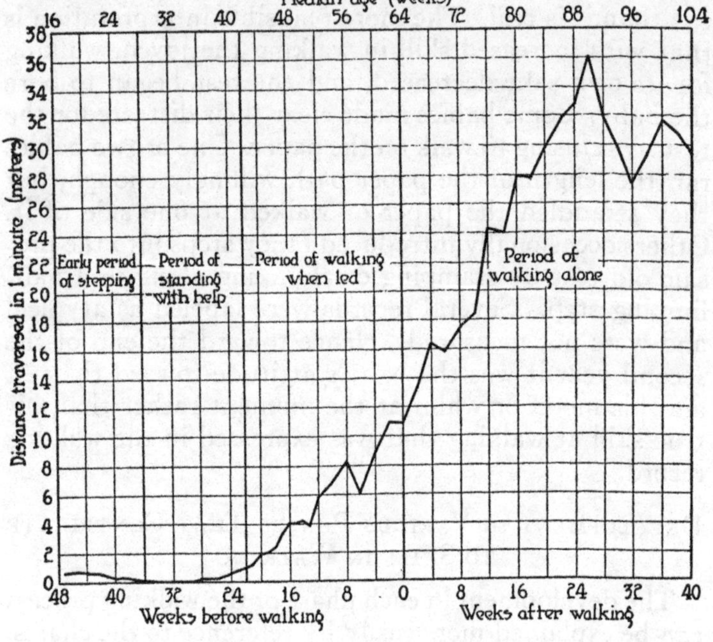

Note that age of walking alone has been taken as a point of reference in computing the medians. For the reader's convenience the "Weeks before walking" and "Weeks after walking" as given at the botton of the graph are converted into their equivalent "Median age (weeks)" at the top. The curve has been smoothed by using a five-point running average up to a median age of 52 weeks, during which period data were collected at weekly intervals. A three-point running average was used for the remaining period, in which data were obtained at biweekly intervals.

usually more sudden than it appears from the chart, but the tapering-off effect came about because of the widely varying ages at which the babies reached this period. For the same reason the curve begins to rise before 42 weeks, the median age at the end of the standing period. The distance traversed increased steadily during the period when the babies walked with help. The greatest increase in distance came, however, after the babies began to walk alone. They reached their maximum distance at exactly 26 weeks or 6 months after they began walking alone, and then according to their records their distance decreased and seemed to approach a plateau.

Number of prints. — The four stages of walking were also clearly shown by the number of prints. The curve for the median prints was smoothed in the same way as that for distance, as indicated in Figure 6. The median number of prints gradually decreased during the early period of stepping, and it remained at about 5 throughout the period of standing. The fact that the median number of prints never became as low as 2 means that the babies usually patted a foot or danced and jiggled enough to make a few extra prints even though they did not traverse any distance. Occasionally there was a slight step backward or sidewise, after which the baby readjusted his balance in the new position. At the end of the standing period the number of prints increased rapidly up to 68 weeks, but after the babies walked alone the increase in total prints was not as rapid as the increase in distance. This has its explanation in the gradual lengthening of the step.

Speed of walking. — Two criteria of speed in walking are possible: first, the distance traversed, and, second, the speed of body movement. For both babies and

FIGURE 6

MEDIAN NUMBER OF PRINTS OBTAINED IN A ONE-MINUTE INTERVAL OF WALKING (SMOOTHED)

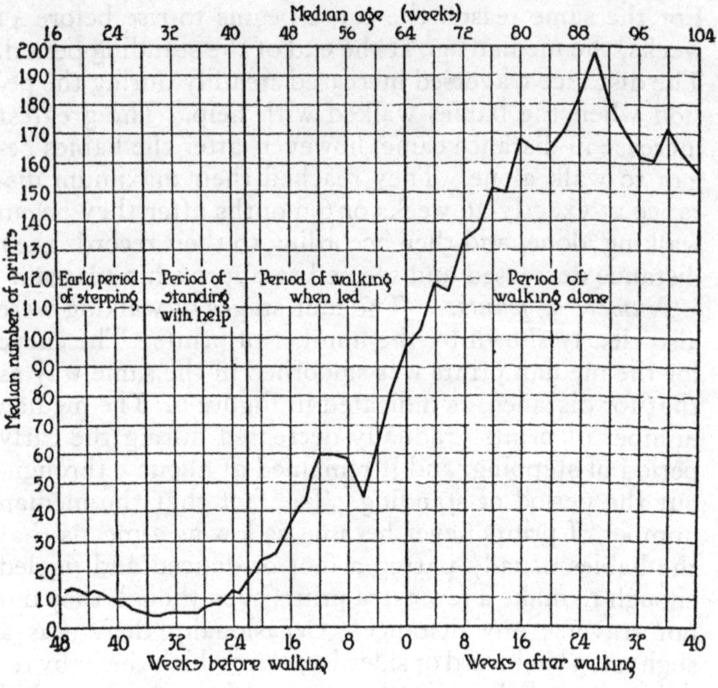

See note for Figure 5.

adults it seems likely that the latter criterion is a better measure of speed. Distance traversed depends both on the length of step and on the number of steps taken, and the length of step in turn depends largely upon length of the leg. Between 18 months and 2 years the babies settled down to a rather uniform rate of walking in which they made about 170 prints and traversed about

30 meters a minute. Four adults, each walking alone briskly on a cold morning, had 145, 142, 143, and 140 footfalls a minute and covered varying distances of 42, 48, 49, and 68 meters a minute, respectively. The first three individuals listed were women and the last, a man.

FIGURE 7

MEDIAN LENGTH OF STEP OBTAINED IN A ONE-MINUTE INTERVAL OF WALKING (UNSMOOTHED)

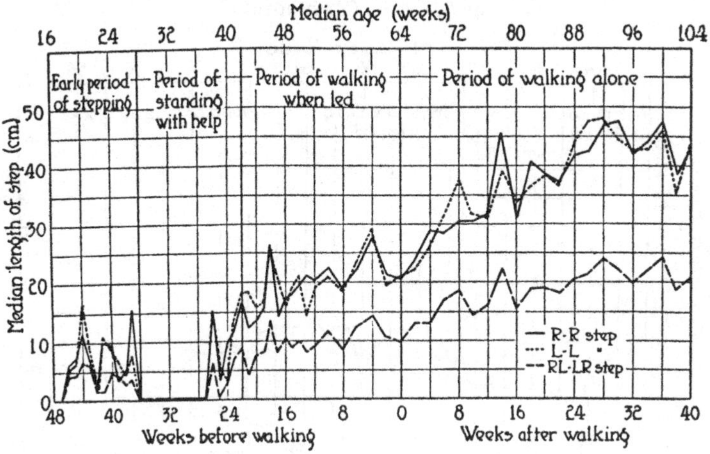

The number of footfalls per minute varied only slightly from individual to individual, whereas the distance covered varied greatly with the height and the sex of the walker. If speed of movement is taken as the criterion of walking speed, the development of walking speed is depicted in Figure 6. These results indicate that the 2-year-old walks somewhat more rapidly than the adult and covers somewhat more than half as much distance. In proportion to his leg length the child probably takes longer steps than the adult. Speed of walking as measured by the number of footfalls increases less rapidly from 18 months to 2 years than does distance traversed.

Length of step. — The babies' steps were short and very erratic during the early stepping stage as shown in Figure 7. When walking began again after the period of

FIGURE 8

MEDIAN WIDTH OF STEP OBTAINED IN A ONE-MINUTE INTERVAL OF WALKING (UNSMOOTHED)

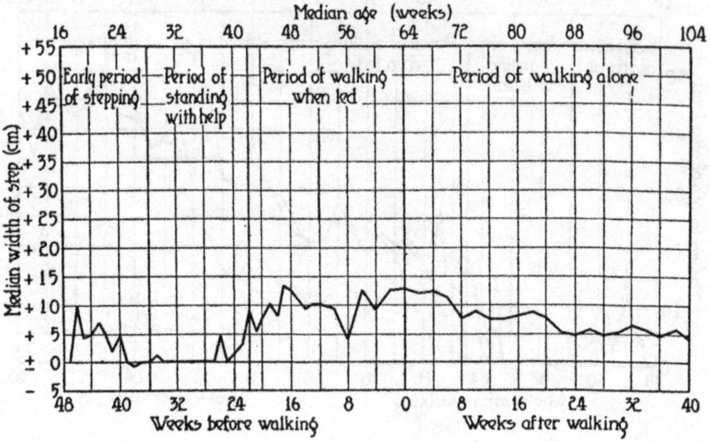

standing the length of step gradually increased till the stage of walking alone was reached, and after this point the increase was more rapid. At about 18 months the step length stopped increasing and remained practically on a plateau during the rest of the second year. There was very little difference between the right-right and the left-left lengths. The single steps right-left and left-right were, of course, only about half as long as the double steps.

Width of step. — The four stages of the walking process in regard to width of step are very clearly shown in Figure 8. The curve definitely changes its direction at the beginning of each new stage. During the early stepping stage the babies placed their feet about 5 centimeters apart as measured by the distance between the

FIGURE 9

MEDIAN ANGLE OF STEP OBTAINED IN A ONE-MINUTE INTERVAL OF WALKING (UNSMOOTHED)

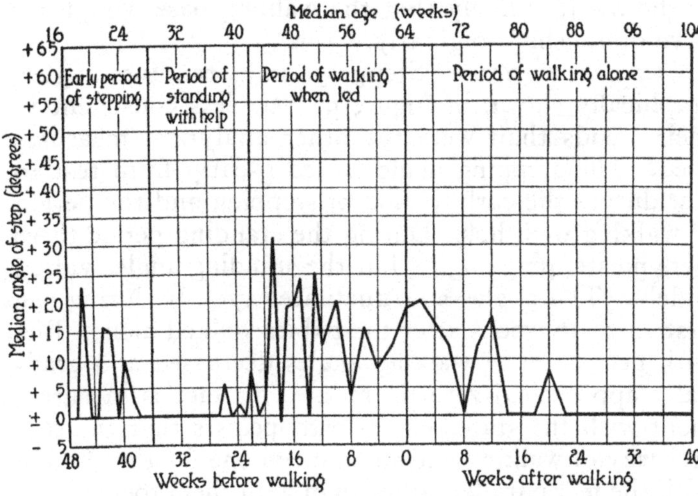

toes of the two feet. At this stage the heels were seldom placed on the ground, and the angle of the feet was difficult to compute. During the standing period the width of the stand was not measured, since standing width is not comparable to stepping width. This is indicated by the gap in the curve. When the babies began to walk with help their stepping width increased rather suddenly and remained at a high point throughout the entire period. As soon at the babies entered the stage of walking alone the width of their step began to decrease and continued in a steady downward trend until the end of the second year.

The decrease in the width of step was occasioned by the fact that babies actually walked with a wide base when they were unskilled but with a narrower base and a narrower step angle as they became proficient. If width of base had been measured at the heel rather than at the toe it is likely that the walking base would not have diminished so greatly.

Stepping angles. — Stepping and standing angles, graphically shown in Figure 9, were less consistent in their trends than were the other analytical measures used. The stepping angle varied greatly from test to test during the early period of stepping and the period of walking with help. During the standing period there were no stepping angles, but the standing angles varied widely. The angles still fluctuated greatly during the first 14 to 16 weeks after the babies walked alone. But with perfection in walking angles decreased and gradually approached zero degrees. This fact is in agreement with the statement of orthopedists that the correct way of walking and the natural one for the child is with the feet parallel rather than with them toeing in or out.

Pigeon-toeing and out-toeing. — In the early stages, however, out-toeing characterized the babies' walking. The number of pigeon-toeing, out-toeing, and straight prints on each record was converted into percentage. Medians of these figures are shown in Figure 10. In the early period of stepping the steps were almost exclusively out-toeing. Out-toeing also predominated throughout the period of walking with help and for 14 weeks after the babies walked alone. Straight steps then became dominant and remained so throughout the rest of the 2-year period. Pigeon-toeing occurred only in a few isolated cases. Only two babies were consistently pigeon-

FIGURE 10

MEDIAN PER CENT OF OUT-TOEING OBTAINED IN A ONE-MINUTE INTERVAL OF WALKING ALONE

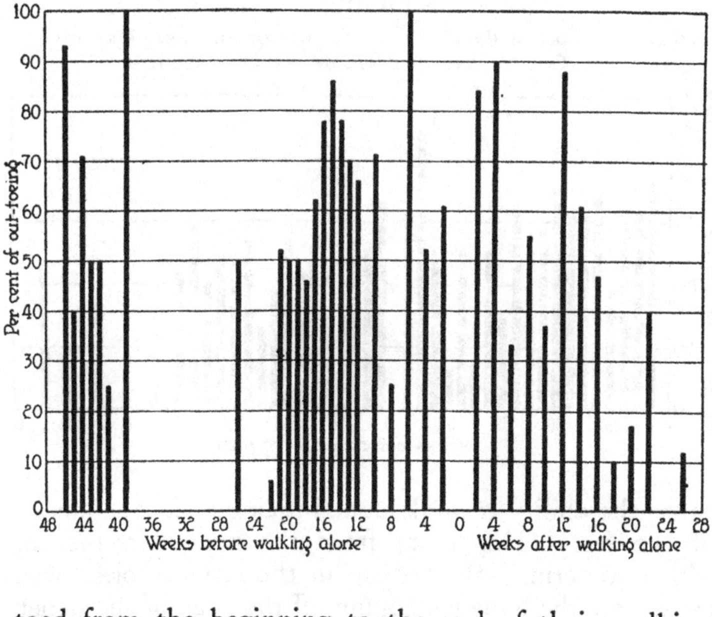

toed from the beginning to the end of their walking tests. Pigeon-toeing was a feature of walking in which individual characteristics of the babies were displayed.

Print sequence. — Another criterion of perfect control in walking is that the prints come in regular sequence, right always following left and left following right. In the early efforts at walking many of the prints came out of sequence. An attempt at a quantitative measurement of this tendency was made by counting every print that followed a print of the same foot rather than one of the opposite foot. The percentage of prints out of sequence was computed with the total number of prints as the basis of calculation. These computations were carried only to the age at which the babies walked alone, be-

FIGURE 11

MEDIAN PER CENT OF PRINTS OCCURRING OUT OF SEQUENCE OBTAINED IN A ONE-MINUTE INTERVAL OF WALKING ALONE

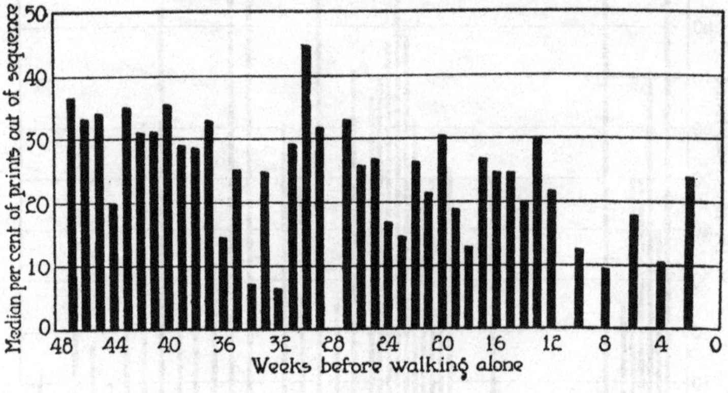

cause the ability to walk alone implies perfect sequence of the feet. Departure from the normal sequence, which sometimes showed up in the later records, was caused by the baby's stepping off the edge of the paper at intervals. About one-third of the prints were out of sequence during the early stage of stepping, as shown in Figure 11. During the standing stage the frequent patting of one foot made the print sequence very erratic. After the babies walked with help their sequence gradually improved, but perfection was reached only when they walked alone.

Patting the foot. — Patting the foot on the paper was a very common reaction in the early ages of walking. It occurred most frequently during the period of standing. This reaction was particularly characteristic of some children and seldom occurred with others.

FIGURE 12

MEDIAN PER CENT OF PRINTS SHOWING TOES ONLY OBTAINED IN A ONE-MINUTE INTERVAL OF WALKING ALONE

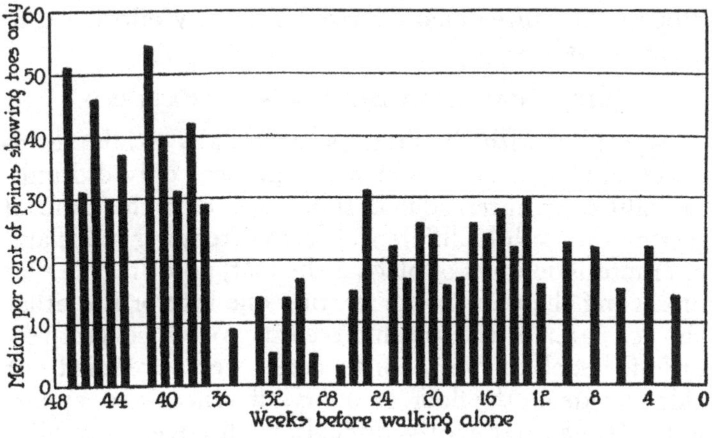

Placing the foot. — Before the babies began to walk with help most of them had characteristic ways of placing their feet on the paper. In the early weeks many of them stood or danced on their toes only. A few made prints in which only the outside margin of the foot was visible, and some stood firmly with their weight on both feet. The percentages of prints that showed the whole foot, those that showed the toes only, and those that showed only the side of the foot were calculated for each record, and the median percentage was computed for each week. The percentages of prints showing the toes only are presented in Figure 12. Throughout the entire period the majority of the babies showed the full foot, and the percentage was particularly high during the period of standing. Toes only were seen in about 40 per cent of the prints in the early period of stepping and in about 20 per cent of the prints during the remainder of the period before walking alone. Prints showing only the side of the foot were of infrequent occurrence, although they often characterized the early efforts of individual babies.

Individuality in the Walking Pattern

Beginning with the first test each baby exhibited individual characteristics in walking. Not only did individualities in interest and skill appear at the time of testing, but subtle differences in the stepping habit and characteristic ways of placing the feet, pointing the toes or curling them under, or patting one foot or the other showed later in the graphic record. When several records for each of four or five babies were stretched out side by side on the floor, striking differences were apparent. It was frequently difficult to discover just what features made each record distinctive. Of course the size and shape of the baby's foot were factors, but apart from this length and angle of step, neatness of print outlines, which indicated that uniform and steady steps had been taken, and character of the print sequence were features that distinguished one baby's record from another's. Assistants who did the detailed measuring of each record became so familiar with each baby's walking foibles that they usually guessed correctly whose record they were measuring before they read the name on the paper. It is not improbable that these individualities of babyhood are the foundation for the slight eccentricities in the adult's walk that enable one to recognize the gait of a friend when his face and figure are still obscure in the distance and the sound of his step before he speaks.

It is worth while, therefore, to describe some of the peculiarities of the walking patterns for each baby, not only in the belief that they will throw light upon the causes for individual variations in walking development, but also in the hope that they will furnish added bits of information that will fit consistently into each baby's mosaic pattern of personality. To give an adequate verbal account of the walking development of each baby would be impossible even if there were unlimited time and space to devote to it. Even in a tabular summary and a brief supplementary description it is possible only to "hit the high spots" and to point out one or two particularly striking reactions for each baby.

The tabulary summary for each baby given in the Appendix should be consulted before the description of his walking habits is read. The summaries and descriptions are arranged in order from the earliest to the latest walker. (See Appendix 8.)

Martin. — Martin was the most precocious walker of the group. From his earliest record at 15 weeks he made forward progress. In the early weeks it is noted that he "pranced as if stepping on a hot stove," and at 27 weeks he jumped on his toes, thus progressing a long way. At 29 weeks he walked across the room in thirty seconds. This baby completely skipped the stage of standing with help. Most of his early walking was done on his toes only. His delight in the test was a joy to the examiners. By 35 weeks he was not only walking well but was stopping to investigate toys on his journey around the room. At 50 weeks he walked alone, and at 54 weeks he walked rapidly without assistance after the bottle of oil. At 68 weeks he began to lose interest in the walking test, sometimes acted bashful, at other times walked off the edge of the paper. At 74 weeks after he repeatedly refused to walk the examiners gave up the test, whereupon he walked up and down the paper several times with apparent pleasure. Now and then he made a good record, but more often he either refused or introduced fancy, atypical steps into the examination. This baby was very muscular and wiry and was precocious in every phase of his motor development.

Carol. — Carol was also precocious in her walking development; with Martin she shared the honor of being the first baby to walk alone. She progressed through the preliminary stages at a rapid rate, remaining in the stepping stage for 3 weeks after her walking records were begun and entering the period of standing at 19 weeks. Her period of walking with help was only 12 weeks as compared to a median of 22 weeks, and she walked alone 2 weeks before her first birthday. After 18 months it was unnecessary to lead her for the walking test. She walked long distances and was very cooperative in the test. In the early record she showed only a slight tendency to walk on her toes instead of on her full foot. Out-toeing steps predominated in the early records, but straight steps predominated at the end. This little girl was small and light on her feet.

Max. — Max was almost a rival to Martin in walking development. Like Martin his record showed no standing period, and he walked alone at an early age. Before he began walking alone he took delight in walking with help, and he tirelessly charged about the house and along the street clinging to one finger of his mother or grandmother. He also was an inveterate kiddy-car operator and raced to the door on it to bid the examiners goodbye. At 49 weeks he refused to walk for the examiner but was persuaded to walk down the paper by his grandmother, who held a bowl of goldfish just out of his reach and called him to come and get them. At this same test his mother reported that he walked alone on the lawn but would not walk alone in the house. His record was cut short by his family's moving from the city.

Virginia Ruth. — Virginia Ruth was a child who could have made an excellent walking record for herself if she had wanted to. She passed through the preliminary stages earlier than the average and walked alone at 54 weeks. But she was by far the most difficult child to handle. At intervals of two or three weeks throughout the entire two years she screamed and refused to walk on the paper. These performances took place at 30, 31, 34, 44, 50, 62, 72, and 90 weeks. In the intervening weeks she often walked well with no objection whatever. At 74 weeks it is recorded that she did not want to walk on the paper but stepped off of it three times, whereupon her mother planted her firmly on the paper, and the examiner led her. At 87 weeks she jerked away, and it required both examiner and mother to get a record. This little girl was not afraid of the paper but, like Matthew, was negativistic.

Sibyl. — The record of Sibyl was very good and not unlike that of Doris. She had entered the standing stage before the records were begun, and by 42 weeks she was walking well with help. At 58 weeks she first walked alone for the bottle of oil. At 80 weeks she developed a dislike for the test, and from then up to 90 weeks she fussed and refused to walk, but at 96 weeks she had recovered from this aversion and walked to the examiner when she was called with no hesitation. Her predominately out-toeing steps became straight after she walked alone. This little girl also belonged in the class of slender children who were light on their feet.

David. — The early records of David were considerably better than for the median, and all indications were that he would be an early walker. He passed through the stepping and standing stages very rapidly and began to walk with help at 34 weeks. His early walking was decidedly pigeon-toed.

About half of it was a dancing and prancing on the toes only, and half of his steps were out of sequence. He frequently patted and pawed at the paper as if he were feeling its smooth surface with the sole of his foot; at 41 weeks he sat down and felt and scratched the paper with his hands. A little later, at 46 and 47 weeks, he walked on the paper as far as the box of toys and then sat down to play in it.

At 54 weeks he walked alone a few steps for his father but refused to walk alone for the examiners. During the following week he toddled about the house alone, his mother reported, until he took a severe tumble on the highly polished floor. The fall frightened him so that he reverted to creeping and did not walk alone again until 60 weeks. His was the only case in which fear set up a complex that definitely retarded walking progress. Even at 66 and 68 weeks he was timid at walking on paper, and as late as 90 and 92 weeks he walked very slowly unless he was led.

Pigeon-toeing, which was characteristic of this baby throughout all his records, represents his chief peculiarity. His left foot was always placed straight ahead on the paper, but his right foot was planted toeing in. He walked on the outer margin of his right foot and curled his little toes under after the manner of a barefoot boy walking on pebbles. This peculiarity persisted to the end of the walking records.

James D. — The records of Jimmy show nothing unusual. He passed through each stage at about the median age and walked alone 4 weeks earlier than the median. His steps were somewhat shorter than average, and his early walking and standing were done on his toes. For several weeks he had difficulty in stiffening his knees, and at 30 weeks he straightened and flexed his knees several times as if he were doing setting-up exercises. At 35 weeks he made his first stand without swaying, but it is recorded that he trembled from the effort. After reaching the stage of walking alone he usually walked well and was delighted in carrying the bottle of oil to the examiner who stood at the end of the path. Out-toeing was pronounced at the start of his walking period, but the angle of his step gradually diminished to zero degrees. He was slender and light on his feet.

HARVEY. — Harvey closely approximated the average in rate of walking development. His two most marked characteristics were wide out-toeing in the early ages, which gradually decreased to straight steps after he walked alone, and very frequent patting on the paper. The total amount of patting done by this baby was greater than that of any other. At practically every test before he walked alone he stamped and patted most of the time. This trait fits in very interestingly with his other behavior; patting and slapping his stomach with good resounding smacks was a very favorite diversion with him before he was 3 months old, and swinging and banging the dangling toys was his characteristic reaction to the choice tests. At 72 weeks he inserted a hesitation step into his walking record; he stamped with his right foot, tossing his head and body to the left side, hesitated, stepped on his left foot, stamped with his right, and so on. Quite clearly this was not his method of walking to get somewhere but merely his way of jazzing up the dull old test. At 78 weeks he strolled leisurely; at 80 he ran to his brother; at 94 he fiddled along, making almost no progress; at 96, 98, and 100 weeks he slid, rubbed his feet on the paper, and refused to walk; and at 102 and 104 weeks he walked well. His record, more than that of any other child, reflects his mood of the moment and his general personality traits.

WINIFRED. — The walking record of Winifred closely approximates the average in all respects. She went through each preliminary stage at about the average age and walked alone at 64 weeks, the average for the group. Her usual step was a little longer than average when she first walked with help, but it was about the average for 2-year-old girls. Like most of the babies her steps were exclusively out-toeing at first but became predominantly straight toward the end. She was usually very cooperative in the walking test and began to walk long distances with much pleasure some 5 weeks earlier than her twin brother, Fred. On two or three occasions after she walked well alone she was timid and refused to walk at all and at other times walked if she were led by her mother but not if she were led by the examiners. This period of timidity lasted only a few weeks, however, and by 98 weeks she not only walked on the paper to examiners when they called her to come but even stood in the examiner's place at the end of the paper and called her brother Fred to come when it was his turn to walk.

Quentin. — Quentin passed through the early stages somewhat more rapidly than the average but walked alone at the median age. During his period of walking with help he enjoyed the test and usually smiled or laughed as he pranced along the path. After he began walking alone he often ran the length of the paper. On one or two occasions he objected slightly to the walking test. He was particularly interested in the foot-greasing process, usually helped with it, and then carried the bottle the length of the paper and gave it to the examiner who stood at the end of the path. At 90 weeks it is recorded that he pretended to grease his feet before the oil bottle was uncorked, and at 100 weeks he greased his toes before the examiner came to help him. At 98 weeks he dropped the oil bottle in the course of his walk and stopped to pick it up before continuing. This baby was of average build as well as of average walking ability.

Maurice. — Maurice's walking record was also about average. He progressed through each stage at the average rate and walked alone at 66 weeks. But he, like Virginia Ruth and Matthew, was a negativistic baby, and the walking test usually precipitated a fuss. During the first year he cried at least momentarily at every test, and at 29 weeks it is recorded that he started to fuss before he was put on the paper for walking. At intervals throughout the second year he fussed and refused to walk even though his mother coaxed him, but at 74 and 78 weeks he almost ran for the oil bottle. At 92 and 94 weeks he screamed and stamped at the test, but after this he walked well and willingly. His refusal at 88 weeks was interesting; when the examiner started to lead him he pulled back and went after the oil bottle that she had left on the floor and that he usually carried on his journey. His mother then put him on the paper, but he fussed and walked in an atypical way. His ability was average, but his negativism prevented the examiners from getting good records.

JUDY. — Of all the walkers Judy was perhaps the most consistent and the most interested of the group. Her stages of walking were very typical of the median. She made the longest single record of any baby, and although she was out-toeing at the start she soon became in-toeing and remained so throughout the two years. In the early records she bounced and danced on her toes. After she began to stand she occasionally swayed voluntarily as if playing seesaw. At 42 weeks she let go of the examiner's hands momentarily. Usually she gurgled, chuckled, or otherwise indicated her enjoyment throughout the whole test. From 74 to 96 weeks at the examiner's command, "Run to S," or "Take the bottle to S," she ran down the paper, laughing, and holding out her arms to be caught and lifted by S at the end of the path. After 96 weeks she walked more slowly and occasionally did a few fancy steps by way of improving her record.

IRENE MAY. — The walking record of Renie May was cut short by her family's moving from the city when she was 18 months old. She was somewhat slow in her progress toward walking; motion pictures of her at 36 weeks showed her swaying considerably when she stood; walking alone began at 66 weeks. She belonged to the group of plump, short-legged babies, who in general walked later than slender babies.

PETER and PATRICIA. — In passing through the early stages Peter was somewhat slower than his twin sister, Patty, and both mother and examiners predicted that the girl would be the first of the pair to walk alone, but the boy at last forged ahead and walked alone 4 weeks earlier than his sister. Both babies bore little weight on their feet in the early tests and did much jiggling and swaying. Peter at 37 and 38 weeks swayed and fell as if in play, repeating the process with apparent amusement. Patty did practically all of her early walking on her toes and progressed in a dancing, bouncing gait. Both babies walked unsteadily at first, the boy with a wobbling gait and the girl with such a wide base that it was impossible for her to keep both feet on the paper. At 79 weeks the records were discontinued when the mother left town for the summer; both babies were still taking short steps. These children belonged to the fat, short-legged group, a fact that may account for their being slow walkers.

WALLEY. — Although he passed through the early stage somewhat more slowly than the average, Walley was only two weeks behind the group when he began walking alone. He was a large, heavy baby and in the early weeks had difficulty in supporting his weight on his feet. He often flexed his legs at the hips as if he were about to sit down but stood thus, leaning backward. After he began walking alone he walked rapidly and made some very long records. At 96 and 98 weeks he had a brief period of negativism during which he refused to walk, but in all other tests he was very cooperative.

WILLIAM FREDERICK. — Fred entered each new stage from 2 to 6 weeks later than did his twin sister and progressed through them at a somewhat slower rate. His records of steps show nothing extraordinary except that in the early period the angle of his steps was somewhat larger than average and about 40 per cent of his steps were out of sequence. He showed no great consistency in out-toeing, pigeon-toeing, or walking straight at first, but the percentage of straight steps increased after he walked alone. His first attempts at walking with help were very clumsy. At two different tests it is recorded that he lumbered along at a bear-like gait, and once he progressed by lifting both feet and swinging by his hands. Still later, on two occasions when he walked well with help, he stamped down the path in high spirits and made such a racket that the examiner jotted down the note, "Walks like stone images in play 'Gods of the Mountain.'" At the end of the period he walked very well. His early clumsiness might be accounted for by the fact that he was a very large baby for his age; he was not only tall, but also heavy. During the second year he grew in height but increased little in weight and thus became proportionally thinner.

DONOVAN. — The records of Don are too incomplete to be very conclusive. Many tests were missed on this baby because of illness and because of a summer vacation away from the city. Although he had reached the standing stage before his records were begun, he remained in it much later than the average. But his standing was excellent; it is recorded that at 42 weeks he surged back and forth and let go one of the doctor's hands. From 54 to 74 weeks he walked well but occasionally screamed and fussed apparently because he disliked walking in his bare feet or because the foot-greasing process was unpleasantly ticklish. Throughout his entire record he rarely had steps out of sequence or stopped to pat his feet. His steps were shorter than the average. Like Fred, Don was rather fat and short-legged, and this perhaps accounts for his slowness in walking.

TOREY. — Torey was outstanding as a poor walker. All of his prewalking records showed him in the standing stage, but his standing was very poor. He did not stiffen his knees and never stood longer than a few seconds. Usually he swung his feet forward, flexing them at the hip, and sat down. When he did stand he touched his toes only to the floor. His mother became very alarmed about him because he was unable or unwilling to put his weight on his heels. At 72 weeks he walked with help for the first time, and since he almost ran he made a very long record. At 74 weeks he walked alone well and thereafter made good records during the rest of the second year. Torey was heavy for his height and had the shortest legs and the smallest feet in proportion to body size of any baby in the group.

LARRY. — Larry was the slowest baby of the group in respect to walking development. The stages of standing and walking with help were longer for him than those for most babies, and each of these stages represented rather poor performance, but when he began walking alone he was proficient at it. In his early tests he made no effort to stand but either drew both feet up and swung by his hands or crumpled up his legs and sat down. This reaction happened occasionally even after he began to walk with help. After he began walking alone he walked with a very wide base. Frequently he walked slowly, but it was often unnecessary to lead him. He enjoyed taking the oil bottle to S. His slowness in walking is perhaps to be accounted for on the basis of his poor muscle tone. Although he was a slender baby and might be catalogued in the group of those that were light on their feet, he was always very limber and relaxed in muscle tone.

MATTHEW. — Mat was one of two babies to build up a serious reaction against walking on the paper. For several months whenever the paper was stretched out on the floor he threw a temper tantrum. Late in the second year after a long period in which the walking test was discontinued he did become unconditioned and walked nicely on the path. The examiners have no explanation for his dislike of the test.

EDITH ANN. — Unfortunately the family of Edith left the city when the baby was 44 weeks old, and her record was cut short. It would have been particularly interesting to compare her with Larry, since in their early records the two babies were similar in that both refused to put any weight on their feet but crumpled and sat down whenever they were held for walking. Both possessed very poor muscle tone, and although they were alert and eager babies their motor skill developed slowly. A communication from Edith's mother stated that the baby walked alone at 66 weeks but that she seemed ready to walk earlier and when she did at last venture forth she walked well. In this respect she was like Larry.

DORIS. — The untimely illness and death of Doris cut

short one of the best walking records made by any child.[2] She had reached the standing stage before her records were started. She remained in this stage 19 weeks until she was 42 weeks old. Her standing records were excellent from the very first. She planted her feet firmly, steadied herself with her arms, and did very little swaying and no patting of her feet. When at 44 weeks she began to walk with help, her record was perfect. She walked for a great distance, steadying herself well; she had no prints out of sequence and no false steps. Had it not been for the subtle onset of her disease it is likely that she would have walked alone before her last examination at 60 weeks. She was slender and graceful, light on her feet, and possessed good muscle tone. Sometimes the examiner lifted her, supporting her in a prone position, with only her abdomen resting on the doctor's palms. In this position the little girl stiffened and arched herself in a graceful curve not unlike that of the acrobatic dancer who executes a dive and is caught by her partner. Until the last few weeks, when the ravages of the disease had weakened her, Doris was greatly delighted by the walking test.

Summary. — Although each baby had individual characteristics that made his walking different from that of every other baby, all the babies had one characteristic in common, namely, a waning of interest in the walking test after they became proficient walkers. To be sure, each baby had his own characteristic way of showing lack of interest. Some were completely negativistic and screamed at the test; others simulated shyness; still others deliberately walked off the edge of the paper; some were distracted by toys; and some improved upon the plain walking test by fancy steps of their own. This lack of cooperation occurred at varying ages with individual babies; it is possible that it marks the dawn of self-consciousness.

[2] This baby died of miliary tuberculosis at the age of 64 weeks.

Significance of the Stages in Walking Development

The question naturally arises as to whether the four stages of walking described above are characteristic of the natural progress of a baby in his acquisition of walking skill or whether they are merely the product of the conditions of experimentation and hence are wholly artificial. In the first place, let it be said that the conditions of testing were not in the least artificial. The foot-greasing was not an alarming process. Indeed many of the babies enjoyed it and often helped to grease their own toes, and only one baby objected, apparently because it tickled. The babies were comfortably supported for walking in a way similar to the one their parents used in holding them erect or in tempting them to walk. The paper path, it is true, did alarm or antagonize two or three babies, but for the most part the effect was transitory. Most of them liked the paper and toward the end of the second year would sometimes help to roll and unroll it or would practice walking on an extra scrap that the examiners did not use. Indeed, the mother of Maurice reported that she found him one day kicking a roll of toilet paper across the room and walking down the paper path as it unrolled.

Even though the conditions of the experiment were simple and familiar it is still possible that the baby if left to himself might have shown a pattern of walking development unlike the four stages described above. There is, of course, no evidence to refute an argument of this sort. Nevertheless, the four stages described do correspond roughly to walking progress as it is usually observed in babies, both by parents and by child psychologists.

The early stepping stage is shown by almost every

baby between the ages of 3 and 6 months by reactions of pushing or patting the feet or bouncing if he is held erect with his feet touching a table or a lap. Gesell (12) includes pushing with the feet as a normative item for the 4-months-old baby. Forward progress during this stage is more or less accidental and usually occurs when the baby is held at arm's length so that he has a chance to make forward movements.

The standing stage is likewise shown by all babies in their normal development. Between 6 and 10 months most babies begin to pull themselves to a standing posture in their cribs or play pens, beside a davenport, or at the mother's knee. They often stand thus, leaning against a support for several minutes. Mothers whose babies begin to stand at an early age frequently become alarmed for fear the child will overtax his pliant bones and will become bow-legged. Sometimes they try to prevent the child's standing, but the baby usually outwits their best preventative measures and stands in spite of the mother's best efforts to stop him. Gesell includes standing with help as a normative item at several age levels.

The baby also progresses to the stage of walking with help regardless of an adult's assistance. Parents find him walking around the edge of chairs or play pen, or progressing along the wall. He also walks by holding to the hand or the clothes of an adult. Walking with help is an item in Gesell's 9- and 12-months tests. During this stage the child becomes proficient in traveling on a kiddy-car, and his method of progression is usually by pushing forward with alternate feet rather than by pushing with both at once. Parents are likely to expect the transition from walking with help to walking alone to take place within a few weeks. Quite to the contrary, this is usually a long, drawn-out period, and the efforts of parents to hasten or retard it are usually without avail.

No one will doubt the existence of a stage of walking alone, and probably no one will question the validity of the rapid increase in speed of walking and in length of step and the decrease in width of step and stepping angle that go with it. These phenomena that accompany walking alone are no more and no less products of experimental conditions than those discovered in the earlier stages.

To doubt that the stages described represent the true pattern of walking development is to go counter to the common observation of parents and psychologists, and to question the truth of the changes in the elements of walking that accompany each stage is to question the judgment of common sense. For in these stages exists the broad general pattern of walking development, and in the accompanying phenomena exist the details of the pattern.

CONCLUSIONS

1. In progress toward walking alone the babies pass through four stages that represent the walking pattern: (a) an early period of stepping in which slight forward progress is made; (b) a period of standing with help; (c) a period of walking when led; (d) a period of walking alone.

2. Speed of walking increases slowly when the babies are led and at an accelerated rate when they walk alone.

3. The length of step also increases gradually during the two stages of walking.

4. Width of step increases until the baby walks alone and then decreases slightly.

5. The width of the standing base and the stepping angles show great irregularity in the early stages. After the babies walk alone the angles gradually decrease and approach zero degrees.

6. Dancing or walking on the toes only is common in the early stages; in the later stages the full footprint is visible on the paper.

7. In the early stages of walking a large percentage of the prints are out of sequence, but after the babies walk alone their feet follow one another in sequence.

8. Pigeon-toeing is characteristic of only two babies. Most of the babies toe out in the early stages of walking, but as they become more proficient at walking their steps become straighter.

9. The babies show many individual characteristics in angle of step, in pigeon-toeing or out-toeing, in patting the foot, and in standing or dancing on the toes.

CHAPTER VI

INTERRELATIONS OF LOCOMOTOR DEVELOPMENT

Two phases of interrelationship among the various stages of locomotor development are worthy of consideration: first, the extent to which locomotor development follows a pattern, stage succeeding stage in a fixed and orderly sequence, and, second, the predictability of one stage from another. Since age was the only measure of proficiency in motor habits, prediction can be made only in such terms.

Consistency of the Sequence of Motor Development

In Chapter III a study of the several skills that contributed to progress in creeping revealed that each separate stage was a fundamental step in development and that every baby advanced from stage to stage in the same order. This sequence was called the "pattern." Similar pattern-like courses of development were discovered for progress toward assuming an upright posture and toward walking alone. This leads one to speculate as to whether the whole sweep of motor development follows an invariable sequence. On the surface such a state of affairs might seem unlikely for the reason that progress toward creeping, standing, and walking goes on simultaneously, and hence a stage that marks advancement in the creeping sequence may coincide with or overlap a stage in the standing or walking sequence. Nevertheless, an attempt was made to discover if a general sequence did hold for all motor development.

The stages arranged in order according to the median age at which each was reached together with the first and third quartiles, medians, and semi-interquartile ranges for each are given in Table III and Figure 13.

TABLE III

THE MEDIANS AND QUARTILES AND SEMI-INTERQUARTILE RANGE FOR EACH STAGE OF MOTOR DEVELOPMENT

Description of Stage	No. of Cases	Age in Weeks			
		Q_1	Median	Q_3	Q
First order skills:					
On stomach, chin up	22	2.0	3.0	7.0	2.5
On stomach, chest up	22	5.0	9.0	10.0	2.5
Held erect, stepping	19	11.0	13.0	15.0	2.0
On back, tense for lifting	19	14.0	15.0	18.0	2.0
Held erect, knees straight	18	13.0	15.0	19.0	3.0
Sit on lap, support at lower ribs and complete head control	22	15.0	18.5	19.5	2.2
Second order skills:					
Sit alone momentarily	22	20.5	25.0	26.0	2.7
On stomach, knee push or swim	22	22.0	25.0	27.0	2.5
On back, rolling	19	25.0	29.0	32.0	3.5
Held erect, stand firmly with help	20	29.0	29.5	33.0	2.0
Sit alone 1 minute	20	27.0	31.0	34.0	3.5
Third order skills:					
On stomach, some progress	17	32.5	37.0	41.0	3.7
On stomach, scoot backward	16	34.0	39.5	45.5	5.7
Fourth order skills:					
Stand holding to furniture	22	41.0	42.0	45.0	2.0
Creep	22	41.0	44.5	45.0	2.0
Walk when led	21	37.5	45.0	45.5	4.0
Pull to stand by furniture	17	42.0	47.0	49.5	3.7
Fifth order skills:					
Stand alone	21	56.0	62.0	66.0	5.0
Walk alone	21	59.0	64.0	67.0	4.0

From both the table and chart it is clear that the medians of some stages coincide and that there is a great overlapping of stages when the middle 50 per cent of the group is taken into consideration. It was impossible to find a sequence of stages that held for every baby. But a certain amount of orderliness in sequence still held; for example, sitting alone always preceded creeping and always followed tensing for being lifted. This seems to indicate that the pattern of motor development, if one exists, is not absolutely fixed and rigid but that it is flexible enough to allow for slight shifts in sequence in

FIGURE 13

STAGES IN LOCOMOTOR DEVELOPMENT

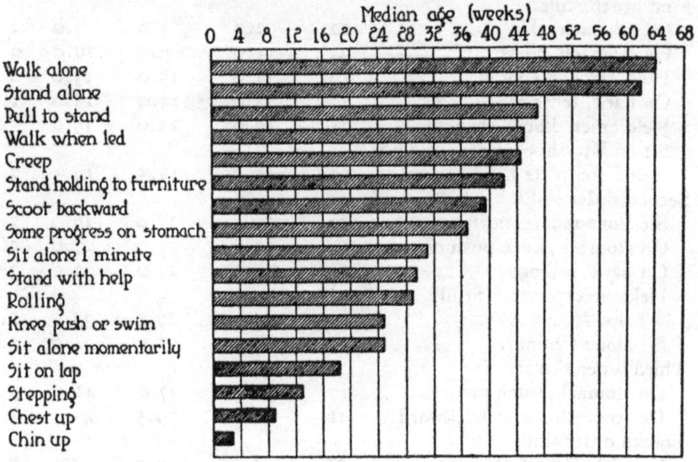

the various stages. The possibility that there were certain groups of stages in motor development that were prerequisites for stages of another group suggested itself.

The sequence of stages for each baby was carefully scrutinized to discover whether the stages fell into general groups or "orders" of development so that there was shifting of sequence in the stages within an order but no transposition of stages from one order to another. The criterion of this was that each order of development be discrete and that all stages within an order become established before any stage of the next order was reached.

Four completely discrete orders and a fifth in which there was slight transposition with other orders were revealed. Thus it seemed that there were five orders of skills in the process of motor development.

First order skills: passive postural control. — Skills of the first order included all those developed by the median prior to 20 weeks of age. They were lifting the chin and chest when in a prone position, making stepping movements, tensing the muscles for being lifted, straightening the knees, and sitting on the lap. At first glance there seemed to be no characteristic that was common to these skills; nothing, in short, that made them hang together except similarity in age. Most of these skills, however, represented the gradual assumption of postural control of the head and upper trunk. Postural control may be considered a passive function as opposed to the active process of locomotion.

A fairly well-defined sequence existed within the limits of this order of motor development. Chin up held first place in 21 out of 22 cases; chest up ranked second in 14 out of 22; stepping ranked third in 11 out of 19; tensing ranked fourth in 9 out of 15; and knees straight and sitting on lap tied for fifth and sixth places. Hence a large number of the babies developed each stage of this order in sequence.

Second order skills: postural control of entire trunk and undirected activity. — Between the median ages of 25 and 31 weeks skills of the second order developed. These skills were sitting alone momentarily, knee push or swim, rolling, standing well with help, and sitting alone one minute. Sitting alone and standing with help are also postural skills, but they represent more advanced control than sitting on lap. Rolling and knee push or swim are active reactions, but they are not very well directed toward locomotion. In this group of skills knee push and sitting momentarily tied for first and second places; rolling occupied third place more often than any other; and standing with help and sitting alone shared honors for fourth and fifth places in order of sequence. Postural control of the trunk was complete and was gradually moving downward to the pelvic and upper-leg region during this order of skills.

Third order skills: active efforts at locomotion. — The two skills that made up this group were progress when on stomach and scooting backward. This group overlapped with the second order skills in one case and with fourth order skills in five cases. It was not, therefore, so rigidly defined as the other orders. The skills of this group were very active and involved great effort toward locomotion with little achievement. Within this order some progress on stomach definitely preceded scooting backward. In this order movements of the limbs gradually became coordinated.

Fourth order skills: locomotion by creeping. — Skills developed at median ages between 40 and 50 weeks involved locomotion. They were standing by furniture, creeping, walking when led, and pulling to a standing position by furniture. Within the limits of this order there was great shifting of sequence. Pulling to a standing position was definitely the most difficult feat in this group. By the end of this order postural control had migrated downward to the lower limbs, and they became capable of either coordinated movement for creeping or of postural control for standing but were not capable of both.

Fifth order skills: postural control and coordination for walking. — Skills of the fifth order were standing alone and walking. These were separated from skills of the fourth order by a long gap and consequently showed no overlapping with any other order. Standing alone either preceded or accompanied walking alone. This order represented complete postural control combined with coordination for walking.

Significance of orders of skills; the pattern of motor development. — It may be noted that each order of skills is separated from the next by a somewhat larger gap in age than separates the skills within an order. Hence some may say that the gap in age is the only factor that makes for discrete orders and that the orders of skills are, therefore, artifacts arising from the method of testing and the way of handling the data rather than facts inherent in the data. In reply to these criticisms be it remarked that although the method of testing was constant, the reactions of the babies were not circumscribed or limited. The observer attempted to record whatever reaction the baby made, and later when the reactions were classified a large number of categories were used in order to prevent oversimplification of the results. If large gaps in age appeared between some stages of development, they occurred because the babies developed no reaction sufficiently different from those that had gone before to be classified under a new heading. It is not claimed that development ceased during the interim between two orders of skill but rather that the development that occurred did not show itself in reactions of a new type.

The development of motor skills is not haphazard but

follows an orderly plan: first, the baby attains postural control of the upper trunk region; second, his postural control moves downward to include the entire trunk region and in addition exhibits random activity little directed toward locomotion; third, he makes active and and vigorous efforts at locomotion, but his poorly coordinated movements meet with only slight success; fourth, postural control of the entire body becomes complete, and the baby achieves locomotion by two or three methods; and fifth, postural control and coordination are combined and he reaches the goal of walking, toward which all of his development has been tending. This represents the *pattern* of motor development. The sequence is simple and logical rather than elaborate and detailed. In its broad aspects the pattern is inflexible, but in its detail it is modifiable to suit the individual capacities of each baby.

Prediction of the Age of Walking

Correlations. — Some indication of the relation between various stages of walking was given in correlation coefficients between various stages. A rank order correlation between the ages of standing with help and walking alone yielded a coefficient of $+.80 \pm .06$ and a coefficient of $+.88 \pm .04$ between ages of walking with help and walking alone. Similarly the coefficient between ages of creeping and of walking alone is $+.84 \pm .05$.

Graphic representation. — The extent of relationship among various stages of motor development is clearly shown in Figure 14. Individual babies are ranged along the axis of abscissas in order of the age at which they first walked alone. Age in weeks is plotted along the axis of ordinates, and bars are erected that indicate the age at which each baby reached the stages sitting on lap,

FIGURE 14

Relationship of Four Stages of Locomotor Development in Individual Babies

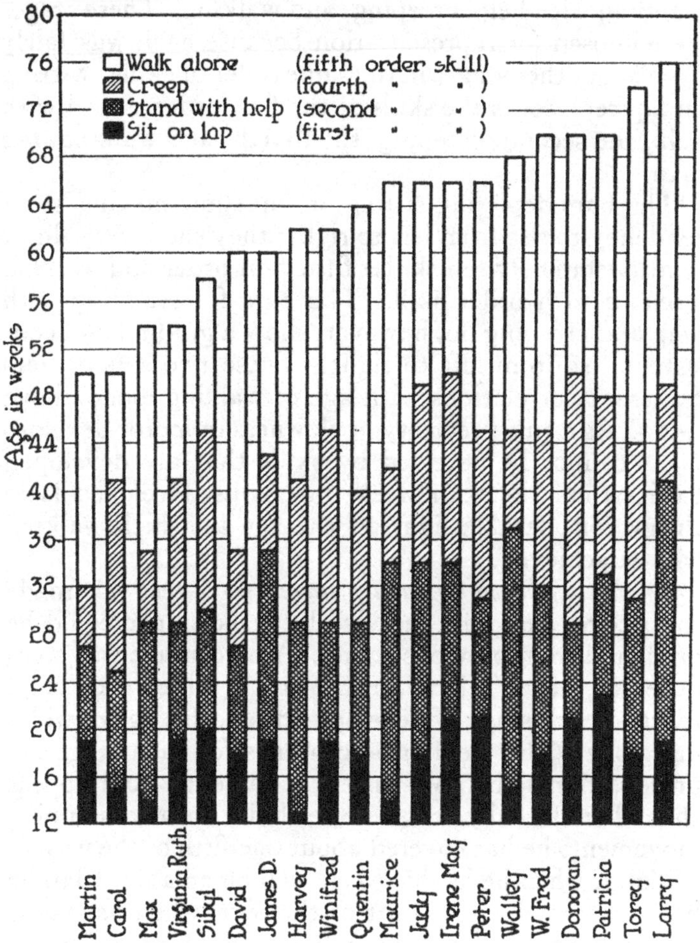

The babies are arranged in order according to the age at which each walked alone. The chart gives a rough idea of the extent of correlation between the various stages. It will be noted that the bars for "Sit on lap" show no tendency to rise from left to right, whereas those for "Stand with help" and "Creep" do rise, thus showing some relation to age of walking.

standing with help, creeping, and walking. These stages were chosen for representation because each was fairly typical of other stages in the same order of skills. Sitting on lap represents the skills of the first order; stand with help, the second; creeping, the fourth; and walking, the fifth.

The bars depicting sitting on lap show no consistent tendency to rise from left to right; they show very slight relationship between skills of the first order and walking alone, a fifth order skill. The bars for standing with help and creeping do, however, show a gradual and consistent rise from left to right. These two sets of bars represent correlations with age of walking alone above +.80. As a rule precocity or slowness in motor development cannot be detected by skills that are developed earlier than the 30th week, but skills developed later throw considerable light on the age at which walking will be achieved.

Prediction based on earlier stages. — A test was made to discover just how successfully walking age could be predicted from previous stages. A percentage was computed of the ratio between the age at which each child reached each stage of development and his age of walking alone. The median percentages for each stage are presented in Table IV. From the table it would appear that when the baby achieves the ability to make stepping movements he has covered about one-fifth of the way to walking; when he is able to sit well on an adult's lap he has progressed 30 per cent of the way; when he stands with help or sits alone he is halfway; and when he creeps he has covered two-thirds of the ground.

The value of these five stages for predicting age of walking varies. For predicting walking age each baby's age of stepping was multiplied by 5. The deviations be-

TABLE IV

THE MEDIAN PERCENTAGES WHEN AGE IS EXPRESSED IN PERCENTAGE OF AGE OF WALKING

Description of Stage	Value in Per Cent	Q	Median Error in Predicting Walking Age in Weeks
Chin up	6.0	±4.0	...
Chest up	14.5	±4.0	...
Stepping	20.0	±3.0	± 9.5
Tense for lifting	26.0	±3.3	±10.0
Knees straight	27.2	±4.4	...
Sit on lap	30.0	±2.7	± 8.0
Sit alone momentarily	37.8	±6.3	...
Knee push or swim	39.2	±3.2	± 5.0
Rolling	45.5	±7.0	...
Stand with help	50.0	±4.0	± 4.0
Sit alone 1 minute	50.0	±3.1	± 4.0
Some progress on stomach	55.0	±5.4	...
Scoot backward	64.0	±5.8	...
Stand holding to furniture	65.6	±4.0	...
Creep	66.5	±5.9	± 4.0
Walk when led	68.1	±4.1	...
Pull to stand	71.5	±4.1	...
Walk alone	100.0	±0.0	...

tween walking age thus predicted and actual walking age were found and the median was computed. From the age of stepping the age of walking was predicted with a median error of 9.5 weeks. Similarly, when the age of tensing was multiplied by 4, walking age was predicted with a median error of 10 weeks, and when sitting on lap was taken as 30 per cent of the walking age, the latter was predicted with a median error of 8 weeks. All these errors were considerably greater than those that arose when one predicted that each child would walk at the median age of 64 weeks. Predictions made by computing walking age as twice that of standing with help and of sitting alone each yielded median errors of 4 weeks.

When creeping age was considered as 66.7 per cent of walking age the median error or prediction was 4 weeks. Hence the age of walking was never predicted with greater accuracy than 4 weeks, but the error made in predicting walking age from later stages of development, such as sitting alone and creeping, was no greater and no less than the error made by predicting the walking age of each child as coinciding with the median.

Summary

In summary, motor development may be said to follow a broad, general pattern in which postural control precedes efforts at locomotion, effort precedes success at locomotion, and some form of locomotion precedes walking. There are many stages in each order of development as outlined above. With rare exception all babies go through each stage, but there are minor differences in the sequence of stages from baby to baby. Precocity or retardation in walking is forecast by earlier stages of motor development, notably walking with help and creeping. Fair prediction of a baby's walking age may be made by doubling his age at sitting alone or walking with help and by reckoning walking age as 3/2 of creeping age.

CHAPTER VII

INDIVIDUAL DIFFERENCES IN LOCOMOTOR DEVELOPMENT

Variability of the Group

From the variability of the middle 50 per cent of the group, which is given in Table IV, it was clear that the age at which each stage is developed varied greatly. The range of the middle of the group was from 4 to 6 weeks even in skills that were developed at very early ages. The later skills such as sitting alone and creeping had even wider limits, and the median range for walking alone was 8 weeks.

Since there was no way of measuring proficiency in a skill, the rate of development at different stages could not be determined. The impression of the observer was that the rate of development was not uniform throughout its course but that it sometimes proceeded at top speed and sometimes was so slow as to be imperceptible. The rapidity with which stage followed stage within a given order of skills and the long periods that elapsed in the transition from one order to the next probably give rough clues as to the rate of development. Certainly the long period between walking with help and walking alone was a period when the rate of development seemed slow.

Precocity and Retardation of Individual Babies

A summary of each baby's peculiarities in walking development has already been given in Chapter V.

Graphic representations of each baby's precocity or retardation in each skill were made as follows. A vertical axis was drawn to represent the median age of development of each skill. To the left of this line were marked off 10 weeks earlier than the median and to the right 10 weeks later. Lines were drawn across the vertical axis to indicate each stage of development, the height of a line from the base indicating the median age of development of that skill. Bars were then plotted at each stage to represent the number of weeks of retardation or acceleration.[1] Samples of these individual charts are given in Figure 15.

Markedly accelerated babies.—By all odds Martin was the most accelerated baby of the group. It is interesting to note that he showed no acceleration but rather some retardation in the development of the first order skills. After the 20th week he was accelerated in all functions, his greatest acceleration being in the functions of creeping and walking. His closest rival, Max, showed almost no deviation from the median in the first order skills. He began to forge ahead of the group in the skills of sitting and creeping, and his greatest acceleration was noted in walking with help. The baby ranking third in acceleration was David. His precocity was not noteworthy in the early orders, but it became apparent in the skills of sitting and creeping. In the latter function his acceleration was as great as that of Max. The best methods of prediction indicate that David should have walked alone at 54 weeks, and in fact his mother reported that he did venture forth alone at this age but that a bad

[1] Throughout the paper the terms "precocity," "acceleration," and "retardation" are only used relative to the median development of the group. They do not imply that arbitrary standards of excellence were set up that some babies surpassed and that others failed to meet, but rather indicate in which direction the more extreme cases departed from the median.

FIGURE 15

CHARTS OF FOUR BABIES SHOWING DEVIATIONS FROM THE MEDIAN AGE IN EACH STAGE OF LOCOMOTOR DEVELOPMENT

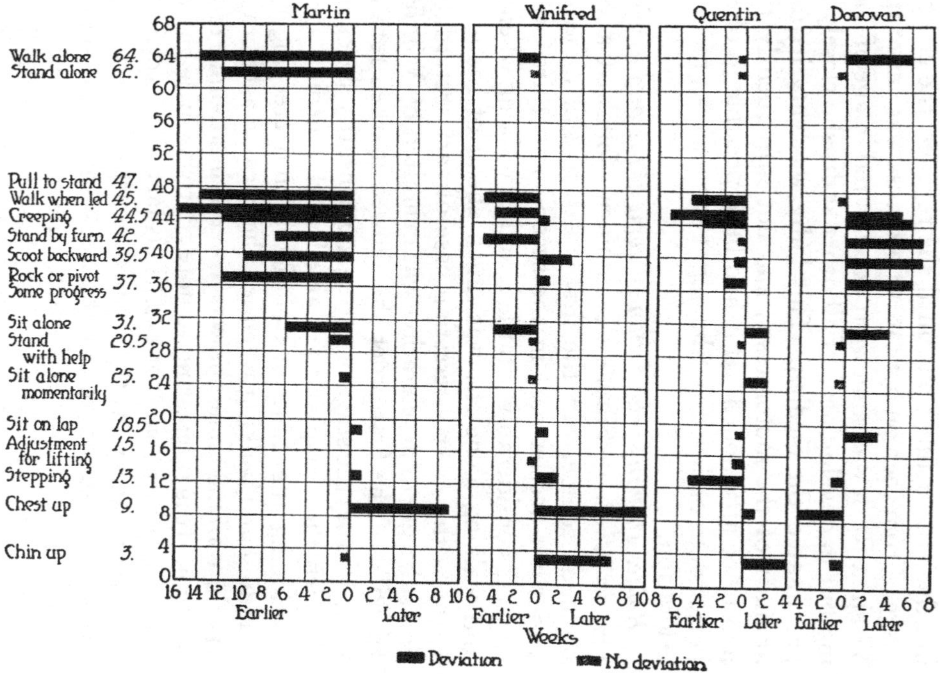

tumble frightened him and set him back 6 weeks in walking development. Although Carol was as accelerated in walking as Martin, her precocity did not show up in other motor functions until she reached the creeping stage. From then on her rate of progress was very rapid. Virginia Ruth was somewhat accelerated in age of walking but in development of all other skills she closely approximated the median. This baby was very irritable at most of the motor tests, and not infrequently they had to be abandoned. If it had been possible to obtain better data on her case, she might have shown more acceleration.

Babies showing retardation in some skills and acceleration in others. — Sibyl's development followed a very tortuous course. In the first order of skills she was somewhat accelerated, in the second and third orders she was considerably retarded, and in walking when led and walking alone she was much ahead of the group. Perhaps the most interesting case of early retardation and subsequent acceleration was exhibited by Winifred. In skills of the first order she showed marked retardation. During the stage of sitting momentarily she caught up with the group and remained at the median age in developing the functions of sitting and creeping. In standing and walking when led she became accelerated, and in walking alone she was 2 weeks in advance of the median. It is interesting to note that this little girl was premature by about 7 weeks. This fact may explain her early retardation. At the age of 6 months she had caught up with the group and at the age of 9 months she had made a place for herself among the foremost in motor development. In all skills but those of walking Torey very closely approximated the median. No retardation in his motor skill was noticed except in the function of

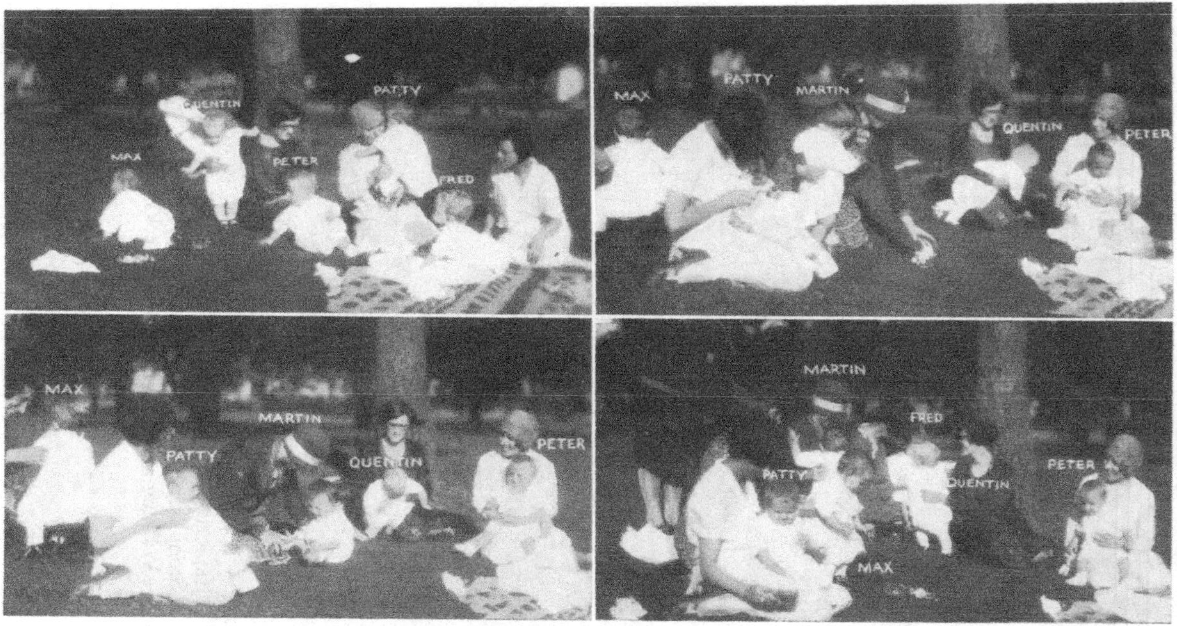

Plate 7. — A Baby Party at 43 Weeks

Individual differences show up clearly when several babies of the same age are brought together. Contrast the active poses of Max, Martin, and Quentin, who are able to creep, with the passive sitting of Peter, Patty, and Fred, who have not yet begun to creep.

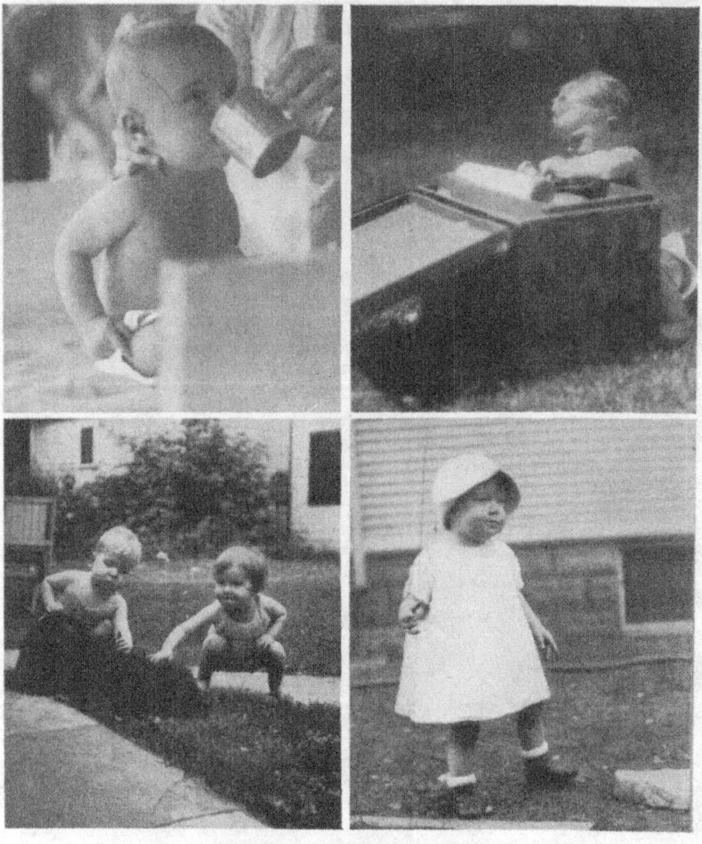

PLATE 8. — BABIES AT PLAY

Upper left. — Drinking like a man: Matthew at 16 weeks. *Upper right.* — Exploring the instrument kit: David at 38 weeks. *Lower left.* — Stooping and squatting: Fred and Winnie at 60 weeks. *Lower right.* — Walking alone: Winnie at 76 weeks.

walking. His great retardation in this skill has already been discussed in Chapter V.

Babies closely approximating the median in motor development. — Six babies progressed at about the median rate in motor performance. Of these Harvey and Jimmy shifted back and forth across the median line frequently but in general were neither retarded nor accelerated. Quentin showed a similar course. In the development of five skills he stood exactly at the median. Peter also approximated the median very closely in all skills, his total amount of deviation being less than that of any other child. Irene May and Maurice each showed only slight deviations from the median, but in general their deviations were in the direction of retardation.

Babies retarded in motor development. — Judy was considerably retarded in all the motor skills involving sitting and creeping. In standing and walking skills, however, she was somewhat less retarded, and her age for walking was only 2 weeks later than that of the group. Patricia showed little consistency in her motor development. In many skills she considerably outshone her brother and even surpassed the median. In the active skills of standing, creeping, and walking, however, she was considerably retarded. The retardation of Larry did not show up until the skills of standing and creeping were developed. In these and in walking he was very slow; at the age of walking he was 12 weeks behind the median.

Don's retardation began at 30 weeks just as the baby was developing skills of sitting alone and creeping. During his 30th and 31st week he had a very severe case of influenza that began with convulsions and continued with high fever for several days. After his recovery from the illness he had a long period of muscular weakness. Furthermore, the mother became cautious about putting him on the floor where there were drafts, and she dressed him in heavier and more cumbersome clothing. She reported that the baby "forgot" many of the skills and tricks in which he had been proficient before his illness. Subsequently the baby grew rapidly and became fairly heavy. Whether or not his later retardation in walking is traceable to this early illness or to his later rapid growth is impossible to determine.

The progress of Fred, 7 weeks premature, was not so brilliant as that of his sister. Like her he was retarded in his early stages, and like her he showed some tendency to catch up. He closely approximated the median ages in the creeping activities, but he was retarded in the postural functions of sitting, standing, and walking. In physical development this boy caught up with the group very speedily. By 16 weeks he was the heaviest baby in the group, and throughout the remainder of the study he vied with Walley for this distinction. It seems likely that his rapid physical growth made for a slight retardation in motor development.

The record of Walley is similar to that of Fred. From the outset he was slow in motor development, his retardation being greatest between the ages of 35 and 50 weeks when the functions of sitting, creeping, and standing were developing. In age of walking he was only 4 weeks retarded. His large size may be accountable for his slowness in motor development.

Summary

Within a group of healthy babies great differences exist in the age of developing motor skills. The reasons for this range cannot be explained on the basis of differences in the babies' opportunities and practice. All the babies had freedom to take as much motor exercise as they liked. One may look to physical differences for explaining differences in motor development; if they fail, the differences can only be explained in terms of predisposition toward motor skill.

CHAPTER VIII

RELATION OF PHYSICAL GROWTH TO LOCOMOTOR DEVELOPMENT

To untangle the complexity of physiological factors that may be related to motor development is an almost hopeless task. Even to discover factors that seem by necessity and logic to bear a relation to motor development taxes one's powers of observation and analysis. Physiological elements that suggest themselves as bearing relationship to motor skill are muscle tone and general health and vigor; anthropometric factors are trunk length, leg length, height, weight, and their interrelations; and probably more important than these are the growth and maturation of the nervous system. Finally, there are factors in part physiological, in part hereditary, and in part temperamental that apparently are involved in all motor development. These are the child's predisposition to good motor coordination, his general store of muscular energy, and his proclivity to expend it.

Of these factors height and weight are the ones most affected by growth. Muscle tone, predisposition to good coordination, vigor and a store of muscular energy, and proclivity toward activity are characteristics more or less constant for the individual baby. Although these last-named factors are incommensurable from birth, they nevertheless form a part of the baby's organization that make him behave as a unit personality over and above the amorphous bundle of reflexes into which his reactions can be analyzed. In the present study these factors seemed to change little with increasing age, and the changes that did occur seemed always to be consistent with the baby's general personality organization rather than counter to it. Since height, weight, and the anatomical location of the center of gravity changed with growth, and since tonus, general coordination, and energy apparently did not, it would seem logical to look to the former for an explanation of the pattern of motor development and to the latter for an understanding of the tremendous individual differences in rate of development.

Anatomical Factors Possibly Related to Motor Skill

Growth of the legs. — It is a well-known fact that at birth the leg length is short in comparison to the body length but that the legs grow more rapidly in the early years, and thus the ratio of leg length to trunk length constantly increases throughout childhood. The possibility of there being a minimum leg-trunk ratio that must be reached before a child can walk alone suggests itself. The anthropometric records were consulted for material on this point. As a preliminary way of discovering a possible relationship between the leg length–stem length ratio and walking ability, the crown-rump measurement, which was taken on a special measuring board, was subtracted from the crown-heel measurement, similarly taken, and the difference was divided by the crown-rump measurement. This method is admittedly crude and inaccurate, for some anthropometrists claim that the crown-rump measurement is the most variable and unreliable of the measures commonly used. The use of the formula crown-heel minus crown-rump divided by crown-rump magnifies the inaccuracy by introducing this erroneous measure into both terms of the fraction. Furthermore, total leg length is not represented by the difference between crown-rump and crown-heel measurements. No single measure of leg length was taken, however, and this difference was used as an approximation. When the anthropometric measurements are analyzed in detail the growth of each child in each feature will be represented by a smoothed curve that has been mathematically fitted to the points. The monthly measurements for each dimension that can then be read from the charts will be more constant than the monthly measurements that were actually recorded. But such refined analysis is a slow process and is hardly worth waiting for, since the chances are that the correlation between leg length and motor skill is by no means a perfect one and that it will not be increased in size nor will it stand out more clearly even if it be derived by a more refined technique. It is hoped that when the data are worked over later these crude preliminary results will be confirmed.

The median of the ratios obtained at each age and also those obtained when the babies were shifted to keep progress at walking constant are presented in Table V. The ratios increased with age in the expected way. By 32 weeks, 1 week later than the median age for sitting alone, the median ratio had reached .55; at 56 weeks the median reached .60 and remained above that point thereafter. When the ratios were computed with age at walking constant they were also found to reach .60 and cluster closely around that point in the weeks just before and after walking. There is no definite demarcation in the ratios to correspond to the different stages of motor development. Active progress toward locomotion did not begin until the ratio reached .55, and walking alone not until approximately .60.

The criticism may be raised that leg length and progress toward walking are related only in that both are functions of age. This criticism is a valid one. It is

TABLE V

RATIO OF LEG LENGTH TO TRUNK LENGTH*

Based on Age		Based on Age at Walking	
Age in weeks	Median Ratio	Weeks before Walking	Median Ratio
0	48.4	62	50.7
4	51.5	58	51.5
8	51.7	54	48.3
12	52.5	50	51.6
16	51.8	46	52.6
20	52.4	42	52.0
24	52.0	38	53.9
28	54.5	34	54.2
32	54.8	30	55.8
36	56.6	26	55.5
40	57.0	22	56.1
44	55.5	18	56.5
48	57.5	14	56.0
52	57.0	10	61.3
56	60.6	6	60.3
60	61.2	2	58.9
64	62.0	Weeks after Walking	
68	61.7	2	57.0
72	62.4	6	59.3
76	64.2	10	63.6
80	62.0	14	61.7
84	63.0	18	63.0
88	67.5	22	65.5
92	68.0	26	64.1
96	63.8	30	65.2
100	66.8	34	65.3
104	65.7	38	68.0

* The ratios were computed according to the formula $\frac{\text{Leg length}}{\text{Trunk length}} \times 100$.

true that medians of the leg-trunk ratios increase somewhat more consistently when referred to time from birth rather than when referred to time from walking. But even so the possibility that the ratio is truly related to walking development is not ruled out.

The importance of the ratio shows up rather clearly in certain isolated cases. The first baby to achieve and maintain a leg-trunk ratio of .60 or above was Martin, who walked alone at the earliest age, 50 weeks. The next three babies to achieve ratios above .60 were Virginia Ruth, Sibyl, and Max who walked alone at 54, 58, and 54 weeks, respectively. Of the five babies to walk alone before 60 weeks, four achieved leg-trunk ratios above .60 earlier than any other babies; the only exception was Carol, a small-boned child, who walked alone at 50 weeks and who ranked eighth in achieving a leg-trunk ratio above .60. The last four children to achieve this ratio walked alone at 70, 66, 74, and 68 weeks, all of which ages were later than the median. In general, the evidence points toward the conclusion that long-legged babies walk earlier than short-legged ones. Proportionate long- or short-leggedness is by no means the all-important growth factor concomitant with walking. The concomitance of the two does not imply interdependence; it may mean only mutual dependence on some third factor, such as age.

Weight-height ratio. — Weight-height ratios were computed for each baby at each age by the formula $W/H^3 \times 100$, weight converted into grams and height into centimeters. The results are shown in Table VI. The median ratios decreased with age in the expected way. Before 44 weeks the median ratios were all above 2.50, but at this age they suddenly dropped about 20 points and did not rise above 2.31 again throughout the two years. From 72 to 104 weeks the ratios ranged downward from 2.00. It is an interesting fact that the first drop of 20 points occurred at the median age for creeping and that the drop below 2.00 occurred shortly after the median age for walking. Individual curves of the ratios showed that the ratios rather consistently remained on a level during

TABLE VI

WEIGHT-HEIGHT RATIO*

BASED ON AGE		BASED ON AGE AT WALKING	
Age in Weeks	Median Ratio	Weeks before Walking	Median Ratio
4	2.52	62	2.56
8	2.60	58	2.67
12	2.62	54	2.62
16	2.70	50	2.68
20	2.60	46	2.72
24	2.67	42	2.66
28	2.58	38	2.67
32	2.53	34	2.65
36	2.53	30	2.59
40	2.53	26	2.51
44	2.27	22	2.55
48	2.29	18	2.58
52	2.31	14	2.57
56	2.18	10	2.26
60	2.14	6	2.19
64	2.10	2	2.39
68	2.19	Weeks after Walking	
72	1.93	2	2.29
76	2.01	6	2.27
80	2.03	10	2.13
84	1.91	14	2.13
88	1.83	18	2.03
92	1.78	22	1.93
96	1.87	26	2.04
100	1.80	30	1.93
104	1.78	34	1.87

* The ratios were computed according to the formula $\frac{W}{H^3} \times 100$.

the first 8 months of life. After that age the ratios all began to descend. The curves for eighteen out of the twenty babies showed rapid drops in the ratio just before or just after the creeping stage; they continued to fall rapidly until the stage of walking and then more slowly up to 18 months, after which they gradually approached a level.

It is impossible to tell whether the decrease in weight-height ratio is a cause, an effect, or merely a related phenomenon of motor development. Perhaps the baby whose weight-height ratio is above 2.50 is so burdened by his excess weight that he cannot lift his trunk from the floor for creeping. But it is just as logical to suppose that his strenuous efforts to creep serve as reducing exercises and that he works off some of his surplus weight in this way. Since the second marked decrease in the ratio comes 8 weeks after the median age for walking, some credence is lent to the latter hypothesis.

When the ratios were redistributed according to age of walking they became less consistent in their gradual decrease. This, however, came about largely because the number of cases was reduced by redistribution. Nevertheless, the median ratio was below 2.30 before walking began.

Again individual cases add to the significance of the weight-height ratios in motor development. Martin, the most precocious walker, never had a ratio above 2.53 during the entire 2 years; at the age of walking his ratio dropped 11 points, from 2.39 to 2.28. The highest ratio for Max, a short, stocky baby, was 2.80 at 20 weeks; a significant drop in the ratio occurred 8 weeks after he crept, and his ratio was 2.30 when he began to walk. David had a low ratio from the beginning; he began creeping at 35 weeks, his ratio at that time being 2.20, and when he began to walk it was only 2.10. One other baby, Carol, was precocious at walking but somewhat slow at sitting and creeping. Her ratio was only 2.60 in the early weeks, but it rose to 2.83 in the weeks between sitting and creeping. It was as high as 2.54 when she began to walk, but within the next 4 weeks it dropped to 2.37. This short, small-boned child proved an exception to both theories of anatomical correlates with motor skill.

Fred and Walley may have been retarded in walking solely because of their great size. Both were tall, large-boned babies capable of carrying great weight. Throughout the entire 2 years they were the heaviest babies in the group. The ratio of Walley remained above 2.50 up to 56 weeks, a high point for babies over 1 year old. Twelve weeks later when he walked alone the ratio was reduced to 2.19 and remained below 2.20 thereafter. The ratio of Fred was only 2.10 at 52 weeks, but it rose to 2.30 at 68 weeks and dropped rapidly to 1.90 after he began walking.

Don and Torey were both short, fat babies. They attained the highest ratios in the group, Don going as high as 2.97 at 8 weeks and Torey reaching 3.11 at 20 weeks. Don, Torey, and Walley were the only ones to have ratios above 2.50 after the first year. At 56 weeks Don's ratio was 2.60 and Torey's was 2.70. Don walked alone at 70 weeks, and Torey at 74. At the end of the second year their ratios were still high, 2.12 for Don and 2.18 for Torey.

The records of Quentin and Larry are flagrant exceptions to the correspondence noted above. From birth both these babies had very low weight-height ratios. Quentin's ratio was never higher than 2.32 and it was below 2.00 at 1 year. This baby walked at exactly the median age. Although Larry's ratio was as high as 2.60 before 6 months, it was reduced to the region of 2.00 at 40 weeks and did not rise appreciably above that point. Nevertheless, Larry was by far the most retarded baby of the group in walking. His slowness cannot be explained on this physical basis.

Maturation of the nervous system. — Concerning the growth and development of the nervous system no data are available on these babies. From the literature on comparative neurology there is ample evidence that development of the nervous system plays an important rôle in the onset of locomotion. This material will be considered in Chapter XII.

Physiological Factors Involved in Walking Development

Muscle tone. — No adequate method of measuring a baby's muscle tone has been invented. Like factors of personality it is a subtle trait that can be observed in a general way but that cannot be scored quantitatively. Throughout this study the doctor estimated the baby's muscle tone at each physical examination by the use of a crude 4-point scale. A rating of 1 point was given for very poor muscle tone and was never given to a well child; a rating of 2 designated tone markedly lower than average; a rating of 3, somewhat under average; and a rating of 4, good muscle tone. The last rating was given most often. Only one child, Larry, was repeatedly given ratings of 2 and after 40 weeks was never given a rating higher than 3. This child, it will be remembered, walked alone at the latest age, 76 weeks. On the other hand, Martin and Max who were the first two boys to walk alone possessed excellent muscle tone from birth. Since the rating of 4 was given in a clinical sense to indicate that tone was up to standard, there was no way of designating tone better than normal. If there had been Martin unquestionably would have headed the list, and Max would have been a close second. The examiners very early nicknamed Martin "young Hercules," and they constantly marveled at his delight in being jumped and swung through the air like an acrobat. He outdistanced all the babies at creeping and walking with help; he walked alone at the early age of 50 weeks and by 18 months he was scaling up the front of a dresser and climbing to the top of a 5-foot wire fence. In his case the 4-point rating for muscle tone was once stretched to 5 points, and to differentiate it adequately from the normal tone of the other babies it should have been rated even higher. The evidence with regard to muscle tone is largely confined to isolated cases, but here it is pretty convincing that muscle tone plays an important rôle in motor development.

Predisposition to good coordination and willingness to expend energy. — There was not even an estimate made for predisposition to good coordination and for willingness to expend energy, but marked differences in both these traits did appear. From the outset Don, Torey, and Irene May were unsteady and a little awkward in their movements, whereas Carol's, Doris' and Sibyl's movements were dainty and full of grace. The babies in the former group walked somewhat later than the median, and those in the latter group walked earlier.

Had the equipment been available it would have been very interesting to have had activity records on all of the babies. The Johnson kinetograph beds provide activity records during a baby's sleep, but there is no apparatus for recording accurately the daytime activity of children and still allowing them the range of the house. The examiners' impressions again have to be taken for what they are worth, although they are supplemented and corroborated by notes on motor play. Martin, who walked at 50 weeks, without doubt ranked highest for delight in physical activity; Max, Virginia Ruth, and Harvey whose walking ages were 54, 54, and 62 weeks would perhaps come next in the order given. On the other hand, certain babies were lackadaisical and lazy. To be sure, each movement counted when they made one, but they did not jiggle and dance and bounce about as much as the babies listed above. Babies who were classed in this group are Fred, Don, Irene May, Torey, Peter, Patty, and Walley, who walked alone at the ages 70, 70, 70, 74, 66, 70, and 68 weeks, respectively. This matter of physical activity will be dealt with at greater length in the chapter on motor play.

Summary

No direct point-to-point correspondence exists between any anatomical or physiological trait and motor development. In general it may be stated that thin, muscular babies and small-boned babies walk earlier than short, rotund babies and exceedingly heavy babies. But in the case of weight it is impossible to decide which is the cart and which the horse. Muscular strength as indicated by muscle tone appears to be an important physical factor in motor development. Proclivity to exercise and interest in gross motor play is much greater for babies who are accelerated in motor development than for those who are retarded, but interest in activity logically seems to be as dependent on skill as skill is on interest. The least that can be said is that there are anatomical trends in development that vary along with the broad motor trends. Individual idiosyncrasies in rate of motor development and in delight in activity, which are relatively constant, probably have their origin in permanent physical factors and in such predisposition to motor skill as may later develop into athletic ability and mechanical skill. Gross motor skill may well be a talent that has its source in genes and its seat in obscure physiological mechanisms, as does musical and artistic talent.

CHAPTER IX

RELATION OF LOCOMOTOR TO INTELLECTUAL DEVELOPMENT

Since the relation of motor to physical development has been discussed in considerable detail, some attention should be given to the relation between locomotor and intellectual development. As yet only slight inroads have been made into the accumulated data on intellectual processes, and the results presented in this chapter are only tentative. Further conclusions as to the interdependence of motor and intellectual skills must await the complete treatment of the data on mental development.

Locomotor Tests in Infancy

In the past child psychologists have been wont to ascribe considerable importance to gross motor development and locomotion as an index to mental capacity. Practically all normative tests for babies under 2 years contain such items as balancing the head, sitting alone, standing, walking, and stair-climbing. Gesell's (12) developmental schedule contains 8 items on postural and locomotor development at the 4-months age level, 6 at 6 months, 5 at 9 months, 4 at 12 months, 2 at 18 months, and none at 2 years or thereafter. The percentage of motor tests at each age is 27, 18, 16, 10, 6, and 0, respectively. Similarly Kuhlmann's (19) tests contain 2 motor items each at 6 months and 12 months and none at 18 months. Tests requiring fine motor coordination, such as block piling, form board, steadiness in reaching, and others are included at later ages, but the locomotor skills that are plentifully used during the early months are gradually eliminated from the examinations by 2 years.

Locomotor and postural development certainly does not stop when the goal of walking is reached. Preschool children go on to master the feats of climbing, standing on one foot, jumping, hopping, and skipping, but not until after they reach school age do they achieve skill in shinning up trees, jumping rope, walking on stilts, skating, and swimming. Consistency with tests of infancy would seem to demand that such items be included in examinations for later ages. Their omission implies either that the authors of tests consider locomotor functions of little importance as indices of intellectual development after 2 years, or that the wealth of other, and presumably better, testing material makes such items superfluous.

Of course there is a possibility that locomotor functions are better indicators of development during the first 2 years when development is going on at a rapid pace than they are after walking, the most important phase of locomotor development, is established. Goodenough's (14) work on the Wallin peg-board tests indicates that, although the reliability of the test drops off at successive ages between 2 and 4 years, the agreement between peg-board and Kuhlmann-Binet test scores is practically the same for the different age levels. In a recent study Atkins (4), using a new object-fitting test with high reliability at ages 2, 3, 4, and 5, found that the test correlated well with the Minnesota Preschool test scores for 2-, 3-, and 4-year-olds, but that it did not adequately measure 5-year-olds. These results tend to show that performance tests begin to lose their value as intelligence tests about the time school age is reached. Something analogous might happen in the case of locomotor development at 2 years. Locomotor skill is, however, very different from the ability tested in performance tests, which measure perception of relationships as well as skill in fine motor coordination.

Paucity of tests of intellectual development in infancy. — The reasons authors of tests for infants have included motor items in the tests are three, all of them depending on the fact that intellectual tests for beings who can neither understand directions nor manipulate objects with skill are very hard to devise:

1. In the very young baby motor development is perhaps the easiest skill to observe. The examiner needs only to manipulate the baby in a few simple ways — to lay him down or to set him up — in order to get a fair estimate of his skill. Nevertheless, motor skills are very hard to score in a simple, quantitative way.

2. The reason for the great scarcity of tests other than motor tests is very apparent. Practically the only other test that can be used with a baby who cannot reach is that of getting his attention and interest centered on some person or object. Degree of interest and persistence of attention are quite as hard to observe and score objectively as are motor functions, and they are usually harder to elicit.

3. Finally, most tests necessitate some motor skill. The baby cannot watch a moving object until he has acquired some control of his head and neck muscles. He cannot reach and manipulate objects when he is in a sitting posture until he has achieved some skill at sitting. Consequently postural and locomotor skills seem to take on importance for intellectual development.

Relation between Motor and Intellectual Skills

Some workers have reported slight positive correlations between age of beginning to walk and subsequent intellectual performance. The highest is a coefficient of +.53 between scholarship in the lower grades and reported age of walking, obtained by Aoki (3) in his study of 53 Japanese school children. Abt, Adler, and Bartelme (1) found correlations of $-.37 \pm .03$ for girls and $-.36 \pm .03$ for boys between age of walking and intelligence test scores. The negative correlation indicates a positive relationship between early locomotion and high intelligence. It seems likely, however, that the lower end of the scale is responsible for these relationships between walking age and intelligence. The average age for walking as reported for normal children by Terman (29) is about .8 of a month older than that for gifted children, but the difference between normal and feebleminded children in walking age is almost 12 months.

In general, the simultaneous observation of mental and motor development in this group of healthy, well-cared-for babies leads to the conclusion that no more relation exists between the two functions in babyhood than exists in childhood and adult life, and that locomotor precocity offers a far from satisfactory clue to intellectual precocity. No data on marked retardation in locomotion were obtained on this group.

Relation of fine motor coordination to locomotor control. — The fine motor skills involved in reaching, grasping, and manipulating objects are related to gross motor development but not to a degree that allows for prediction in individual cases. A correlation of $+.42 \pm .12$ was found between age of reaching and grasping an object and the age of walking. Two babies who reached and obtained objects at a very early age were Walley and

Max, the former retarded in walking, the latter accelerated. Many other instances could be cited, all of them tending to show that use of the arms and hands in reaching is a different matter from maintenance of postural control and locomotion. With plenty of support for his trunk the baby is able to direct the motions of his smaller muscles with ease and skill, compared with the awkwardness of his attempts at locomotion.

Slight relation between early and later motor development. — In Chapter VI it was pointed out that motor skills of the first order, head-lifting, sitting on the lap, and others were only slightly related to the later motor skills of sitting alone, creeping, and walking.

Effect of distractibility of active babies on intellectual test scores. — In this study it often happened that the two babies who were most precocious in motor development did very poorly on the psychological tests. The latter tests consisted chiefly in manipulating simple toys, piling blocks, opening boxes, and looking at pictures. For such tests the baby sat in his high chair, on the examiner's lap, or on the floor. Such sedentary tasks gave the active baby no thrill. Usually his health and high spirits could not be curbed for the test, and he abandoned the toys for the more active pursuits of standing in his high chair, wriggling off the examiner's lap, or creeping away. Such lack of interest in intellectual tests does not necessarily imply inability but does give active babies poor scores.

Vocalization and motor development. — An interesting relationship, which will be gone into more fully in a later paper, is that between vocalization and motor development. In the very early weeks it was noted that many babies began to coo and babble shortly before they began to reach. While the reaching act was being perfected their vocal play was very much diminished. It reappeared just after reaching was well established and was again discontinued while the baby was perfecting his skill at sitting. Another increase in jabbering took place before the baby walked. A few babies who were slow at walking were great "talkers" to judge by quantity rather than quality of speech. Walley and Judy developed large vocabularies and spoke more fluently than did most of the babies. Fred's steady flow of speech was largely incomprehensible at first, but it apparently had meaning for him, and he used his linguistic inventions so consistently that he soon made himself understood. Don incessantly sang and jabbered in conversational tones, a jargon wholly without meaning but uttered in long, many-syllabled sentences with perfect inflection. In tonal quality alone his conversation comprised matter-of-fact remarks, philosophical comments, queries, commands, requests, and exclamations; after each he awaited the appropriate reply of an adult.

The vocalization of Martin stands in vivid contrast to that of the slow walkers. He was a child of few words. He could and did talk comprehensibly when he was urged and questioned, but his spontaneous vocalizations were few and were more likely to be shouts of joy at manipulative tests or grunts of protest against sitting down to look at pictures. Two characteristic and interesting expressions of his were "Ah know, ah know" when he was given the form board, which he manipulated with perfect skill, and "me vill" at being asked to run errands. Activity was bespoken both in his expressed thought and in his use of verbs; complacent naming of objects played no part in his conversation.

The substitute nature of the speech response is very clearly illustrated by these observations. The baby who cannot act effectively takes it out in talking, it would seem, just as the adult does.

Relation between score on intelligence tests and age of walking.—The *IQ*'s as computed on the Minnesota Preschool Test that was given at 18 months were correlated with the ages of walking. The 18-months test score was used instead of the 2-year score because the former age was nearest that of walking. The correlation on seventeen cases proved to be $+.28 \pm .14$. Although little significance can be attached to a correlation on so few cases, it confirms the general findings of others that a small but positive relationship exists between motor and intellectual skills.

Summary

A very small relationship exists between locomotor skill and intellectual attainments in the baby, a relationship too small to allow for prediction in individual cases. Locomotor precocity, such as walking at an early age, certainly should not be used as a single criterion for predicting superior intelligence, and motor retardation should not be used to forecast subnormal intelligence unless it is so great as to clearly indicate a pathological inferiority, in which case other supporting evidence of mental retardation would hardly be lacking. Although locomotor items are not included in developmental or "intelligence" tests for children beyond two years, it is possible that they are useful supplementary items in the earlier scales. It is the author's opinion, however, that, because of the difficulty of scoring locomotor items and because of the inconsistency of including them in tests at early ages and excluding them at later ages, authors of tests for babies should make an effort to replace the motor items with other material.

CHAPTER X

LOCOMOTOR PLAY OF BABIES UNDER TWO YEARS

Locomotor play, as the term is used in this chapter, refers to any gross motor activity in which the baby indulged at any time during the examinations other than at the motor tests and also any gross motor behavior reported by the mother. No pretense is made that complete and accurate records of play activities were obtained in this way, but it is believed that there is a fair sampling of each child's play. Certainly a wealth of material was gathered, and a detailed account of it would be voluminous. Only the essential features of the data will be pointed out, namely the extent to which motor play followed the pattern of motor development and the extent to which it expressed each baby's motor skill and his delight in activity.

CONFORMITY TO THE GENERAL PATTERN OF LOCOMOTOR DEVELOPMENT

All the play responses for each baby were sorted into five groups according to the order of development in which the play activity occurred. Thus the babies were equated in motor skill rather than in age. A sixth group was made on the age basis and included all play responses of babies older than 18 months. The essential features in each order of skills will be discussed.

Play Accompanying First Order Skills

Skills of the first order, as described in an earlier chapter, were those of lifting the head, tensing the muscles, early stepping, and sitting on an adult's lap. They were called the passive postural skills and in general they were all developed by 20 weeks. The gross motor play that accompanied these skills was rather meager.

The reactions noted were merely variations of sitting when propped or held, stepping, and turning from back to side. The twins, Fred and Winifred, leaned and reached for each other's toes when they were propped up by pillows facing each other. Bouncing and waving in excitement were manifested by two babies, lifting the head by one, and reaching for their toes by four. Two babies were observed to put the soles of their feet together as if to pat-a-cake with them. Frequently a baby whetted the soles of his feet together when he was struggling to reach a toy. Two babies lifted the trunk slightly for the tapeline to be moved when they were lying on their backs for measurement of circumference. One active baby attempted to slide off the examiner's lap by keeping his knees straight and lifting his buttocks. Another baby stepped with his left foot when he was held erect and thus went around in a circle.

Perhaps one reason for the limited repertoire during the first order skills was that eye-hand coordination was developing at the same time. Much of the baby's play consisted in reaching for objects, and motor exercise was largely confined to wiggling and kicking more or less at random. Motor play of this period seemed to be largely for the sake of exercise rather than for the enjoyment of the activity.

Play Accompanying Second Order Skills

The development of skills of the second order, rolling and sitting alone, was accompanied by many motor activities of great variety. The tendency was for play to lose its random hit-or-miss character and to become somewhat organized, although it was not necessarily directed toward an end. Now and then a baby learned to play a motor game with an adult and played it according to the adult's rules. Most of the play of this period involved sitting or rolling. At this time the baby, like the pure art-for-art's-sake artist, was a pure player, playing for play's sake.

Playing with toes. — The major sport of the age when second order skills were developing was playing with the toes. Twenty babies in the group were observed in toe-play during this period as contrasted to four babies in the preceding and two in the following periods. Playing with the toes had two sets of rules, according to whether the baby was lying or sitting. If the baby were lying on his back, he usually waved his legs in the air, clasped his arms under his knee and brought his foot up to his mouth, perhaps lifting his head and shoulders to get his mouth somewhat nearer the wiggling toes. Sometimes he simply lay with feet in the air, fingering his toes; frequently when he had a firm grasp on his feet he rolled to the side.

It has already been mentioned that in a great deal of the early sitting the baby leaned far forward. This brought head and hands in close proximity to feet, and the baby seized the opportunity to get more intimately acquainted with his fascinating lower digits. In playing with his toes while lying down he brought his toes to his mouth, and while sitting, he brought his mouth to his toes. The former gave exercise in leg-lifting, the latter in trunk-bending.

Bouncing. — Bouncing was also a favorite diversion of babies from 6 to 8 months of age. The babies greatly enjoyed bouncing in canvas swings, which hung by springs from the ceiling. But springs were not needed to keep the babies bouncing; they bounced and waved when they were sitting on the floor, in their high chairs, or on an adult's lap. Rocking in the sitting position has already been described. Scrubbing the heels on the floor and excited waving of hands expressed many babies' eagerness to be picked up, given a toy, or fed. One baby developed a habit of pouncing cat-like on a toy that was put on his high-chair tray.

Squirming, head-shaking, leaning. — As proficiency in sitting increased the baby turned around in his high chair, leaned over its arm to look for fallen toys, tried to slide out of the chair or off the examiner's lap, lifted the chair tray with his feet, leaned to look up at the squeaking spring of the baby swing, and did a great deal of squirming. Some babies shook their heads very vigorously as if in negation, but apparently they did it for the sake of the head motion. One baby lay on his back, his feet in the air pedaling as if he were riding a bicycle; another put his feet together as if to pat-a-cake. Patting the hands was a frequent play activity at this age.

Dancing, pulling to stand. — Dancing, jiggling, and bouncing when held in the upright postures were also frequent at this age. Some babies enjoyed pulling to a standing posture when an adult held their hands only. Three babies seemed to use the soles of their feet for tactile sensations. One rubbed his feet on the walking paper as if to feel it; others rubbed the feet with a cloth or with their stockings.

Cooperative motor games. — Several mothers taught their babies games during this period. Most of these games, pat-a-cake and others, involved fine motor coordination and will be taken up later under that topic. Peeka-boo was sometimes played by the baby's dragging a blanket over himself and kicking it off and sometimes by the baby's rolling over to hide and then suddenly flopping back at the words peeka-boo. One mother utilized the rocking response in the game "Draw a bucket of water for the farmer's daughter." Mother and baby held hands and swayed back and forth to the rhyme. Another baby responded to the command, "Rock-a-bye baby," by rocking back and forth on her mother's lap. She also tried to imitate her father's dancing capers. "This little pig went to market" was a favorite game during this period when the babies' interest in their toes was at its peak; they often cooperated in the game by holding up the "little piggies" for their mothers to tweak and kiss. One baby invented a game of bouncing and hallooing to "scare" his parents, who responded with a jump and a squeal that set the baby giggling. In all these games baby and mother cooperated in making out the rules of the game. Probably baby began rocking or playing with his toes, and mother systematized the acts and suited them to words.

Play of the Third Order Skills

The active effort toward locomotion that characterized the third order skills was very naturally accompanied by active play. Excited kicking, scrubbing the heels, bouncing in the bed and to music, leaning over the chair arm or carriage, and some playing with toes persisted, as well as rolling on the floor or off the bed, turning over in the bath, or playing peeka-boo. New reactions were turning and twisting in the crib, holding to the bars and pulling to a sitting posture, strenuous efforts at crawling for a toy, rolling about in a sitting posture, and getting up on hands and knees to surge back and forth. Some tried to stand and a few succeeded in getting to an upright posture in the crib. One baby tried to imitate jumping by giving a bounce or lunge in the sitting posture. Others began to dance and jiggle when they were held upright for walking. During this stage play was still activity per se.

Play Activity in Fourth Order Development

The development of locomotion brought with it a remarkable increase in the amount and diversity of play. Motor toys began to be used with skill. The most interesting change, however, was that as soon as the baby could move about under his own steam his activity became directed toward a goal and was not indulged in exclusively for its own sake. He used his motor skills to serve his needs, needs usually limited to getting a toy or at most to creeping in the direction of food or water. Activity became a means to an end rather than an end in itself.

Sedentary play. — Play in the sitting posture was about the same for this period as it had been for the two preceding periods. The babies sat and kicked or scrubbed their feet in excitement or expectation, bounced in glee, sat rocking or patting the feet together, on rare occasions played with their feet, sometimes scooted over on the floor or couch to make room for another person, lifted the high-chair tray with the feet, leaned over the edge of the carriage, rocked in a chair or rocking horse, leaned or leaped forward in the sitting posture, or sat shaking the head or swaying to a jazz tune.

Climbing and standing. — Climbing and standing play, aside from that which occurred in response to the tests, was usually activity of the play-for-play's-sake type. Furniture, persons, and the baby's own safety were sacrificed to this great urge to climb. Climbing to stand in the high chair and often rocking it to a downfall, standing in the carriage and sometimes tumbling out, climbing by the bars of the crib and begging to be lifted out were the more spectacular stunts of this age. Climbing to stand by furniture and by persons was a safer process and just as universal. Scrambling to stand on an adult's lap there to poke at eyes and nose, snatch off spectacles, and entangle chubby fingers in stray wisps of hair delighted babies at this stage. Two babies scaled adults who were standing, sometimes shinning up father's legs, sometimes holding mother's hands and walking up her as a lineman walks up a telegraph pole. One baby crept up the tongue of his express wagon and seated himself for a ride. Several began to climb on and off low stools and boxes and to go upstairs on hands and knees during this versatile period.

The standing and walking of this period were done only with the support of furniture or with the aid of an adult. Weeks before he was able to walk alone one baby descended from his perambulator during one of his daily rides and walked down the street pushing the carriage. Some walked a chair about the room using it as a prop. Many walked about freely on a kiddy-car. A few more precocious walkers charged about the house in quest of toys, leading an adult or child for support. For the most part, however, walking was done for exercise only. When the baby really wanted to go somewhere he resorted to creeping. Squatting and rising again to a stand or squatting for several minutes was an interesting adjunct to standing.

Creeping. — Creeping, unlike climbing, was a reaction laden with purpose. During the examinations babies crept to get more interesting toys, to show a prized plaything to mother, or merely to get away from the test situation. In the ordinary day's play creeping served the end of getting to an adult for help in trouble, seeking mother for comfort and sympathy, and following children around at play. Some tried to creep carrying large objects with them, and many crept shoving toy trains or carts along the floor in front of them.

Toys for motor play. — Kiddy-cars of one sort or another, particularly those having a railing to prevent the baby from falling, were much used and greatly enjoyed by these babies. When they first learned to propel these toys they usually went backward instead of forward. Later they careened about the house at top speed, guiding the little cars around furniture and traveling through open doors. Babies of this age knew no danger, and their headlong speed sent two young drivers jolting down the cellar steps. One baby learned to walk around the house in a walk-about. Swings were outgrown by this period, and high chairs were not enjoyed as they had been, the reason being of course that these toys were too confining for the baby and limited his activity too much to please him.

Moving furniture. — During this period some babies discovered that they could move furniture and evidently took great pride in this display of strength. For one examination the baby was seated at a small table, usually a card table. This test involved looking at pictures and magazines, a pursuit in which the more active babies took no pleasure. But instead of throwing away the pictures they shoved table and all from them, sometimes using their hands and sometimes their feet. One baby disliked open doors, and he hitched about the house pushing them shut. Another invented a game of holding and throwing a pillow. One baby moved his little chair under the light switch and climbed up to turn on the

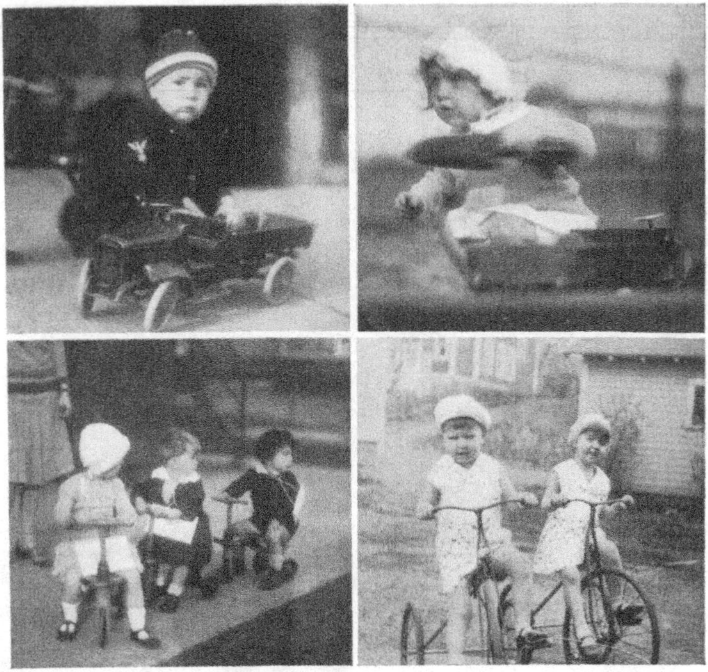

PLATE 9. — MOTOR TOYS

Upper left. — Truck for riding or hauling: Harvey at 2 years. *Upper right.* — Shovel and sand: Sibyl at 2 years. *Lower left.* — Kiddy-cars for 2-year-olds: Judy, Larry, and Maurice. *Lower right.* — Tricycles for 3-year-olds: Fred and Winnie at 3½ years.

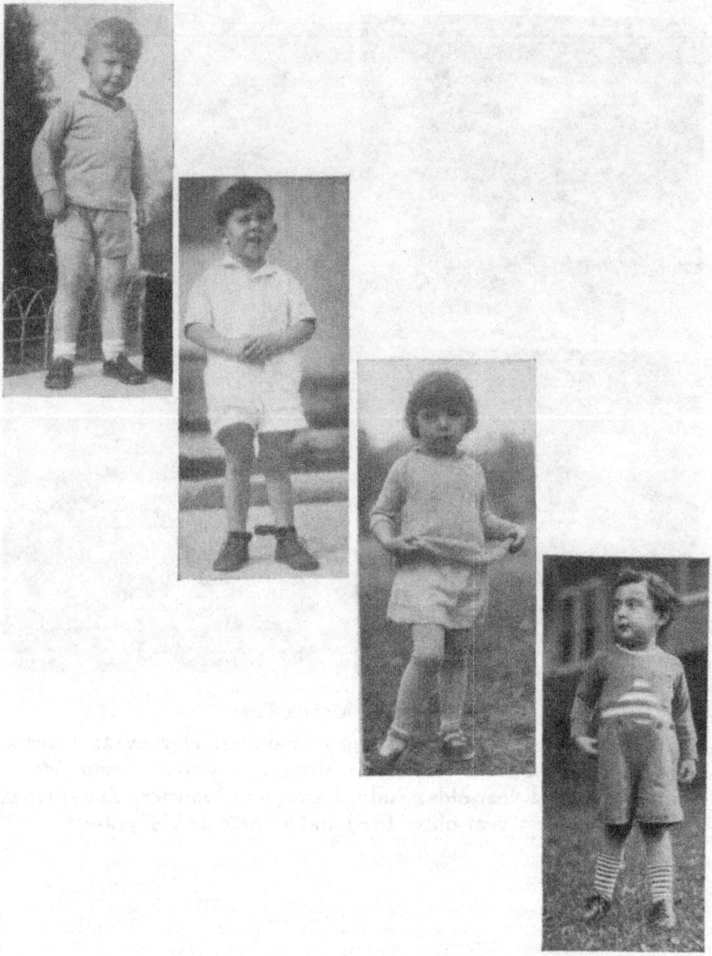

Plate 10 — The Babies Grow Up

From left to right. — Torey, James, Virginia Ruth, and Maurice at 3 years.

light. During this stage he was the only baby to use furniture as a tool for getting a desired object.

Play during Early Walking Period

Once walking began, creeping as a means of locomotion was practically abandoned, although it often occurred in purely motor and in dramatic play. Most of the play of this period consisted in perfecting and varying the walking and climbing activities and in mastering the common household furniture.

Variations in walking. — As soon as walking had become the method of getting around the house it began to be adorned with frills according to each baby's fancy. Some strutted and swaggered about the rooms, stopping perhaps to preen before a mirror; some walked upright on the knees; and two or three walked after the examiners carrying their satchel. Many walked or ran to greet the examiners and followed them to the door when they left, reactions that in themselves hardly deserve mentioning but that indicate that the weekly visits were a joy to both the experimenters and the babies.

Shortly after walking was established, running began. This sport was indulged in chiefly for the pleasure derived from it. Being chased by or chasing an older child or an adult was a frequent variation.

Climbing. — Climbing at this age really got the babies somewhere. They climbed not a few steps but the entire stairs; they climbed not to stand beside but to stand on chairs, davenports, and beds; and they soon learned to scoot down the stairs or down from furniture as well as to climb on it. They discovered that chairs were useful tools for climbing to a sideboard or table after some coveted object that had been put away from meddlesome fingers.

Mastery of furniture. — By degrees the household furniture took on the same values and began to play the same subservient rôle in the life of the baby that it plays in the life of adults. In the creeping stage furniture was the baby's all-but-human helper, his rod and his staff, as it were, and he treated chairs, beds, and sofas in particular with considerable infant deference and respect. The upholstery was patted and clung to almost as was the mother's dress. But at the advent of walking and climbing, furniture became objects to be sat upon, jumped and bounced on, used for tools, and thoroughly exploited. Drawers were opened, doors were opened and closed, even windows were lowered, and every nook and cranny of the house was explored.

Persistence of earlier activities. — Not all of the old tricks were abandoned when walking began. Rocking and bouncing were often indulged in, and now and then interest in the toes was revived. The babies still sat on adults' laps, but they scooted off and climbed on again at will. This was an age of almost complete motor freedom with complete absence of responsibility, for parents gave the babies the run of the house, at the same time surrounding them with safeguards and protection and not yet imposing upon them limits as to scope of activity or punishing misdemeanors.

Motor Play from 18 Months to 2 Years

The babies were allowed to run untrammeled and untamed for only a few weeks. Long before the second year the parental screws began to come down on them, and they were forced to moderate their motor play and to take on some of the motor responsibilities of childhood. They no longer went scot-free after meddling or running away. Errand running — simple duties such as bringing father's slippers and taking soiled clothes to the hamper — was imposed on them. Naturally the child began to take on the motor ways of older children and adults and to do the things that he saw being done. Walking, running, and climbing continued to improve, and dancing was added to the repertoire.

Imitative play. — Imitative and dramatic motor play began about this time. The children, with a few suggestions from older brothers and sisters, were "choo-choos," "bears," or "humpty-dumpty." Some mimicked their parents' walk or crossed their legs in manly fashion. Four children at this age lay down on their stomachs to look at picture books or to write. This flat-on-the-floor, heels-in-the-air position is the stock illustration for the child bookworm, and it is certainly a favorite posture with the 10-year-old for reading and doing sums. Since all the babies who lay down to "read" or "write" were those who had brothers or sisters in the grammar grades, it seems likely that the babies took the older children as their models.

Motor expressions of shyness. — Curbed by a few taboos, the babies began to take on consciousness of self, and much of their shyness and boredom was expressed in motor terms. Reverting to playing with toes or shoes was a favorite way of showing boredom or shyness. The baby would sit with bent head and eyes and with an air of absorption to avoid meeting an adult's gaze. Drumming the heels in a regular tattoo was another way of filling up time until something more interesting happened. Putting his head down and then looking out coyly between his legs or under his crooked arm was the way one baby both expressed shyness and made a bid for attention. Lying down on the floor, kicking and screaming, or throwing a tantrum according to the best authorized versions were some babies' reactions to limitations of their freedom.

Patterns of Motor Play Summarized

The outstanding fact about motor play is that babies play at the level of their motor ability and strength and not below or above it. In their play they exercise newly acquired skills and rapidly abandon those they have outgrown. It is safe to say that the babies never spontaneously try anything that they are not perfectly competent to do. Unlike adults they do not overtax their powers, and parents are probably safe in allowing the baby to do whatever he wishes.

This does not mean, of course, that the baby will not roll out of bed, tip over his high chair, or tumble down the stairs. He is heedless of danger because he does not know the consequences, and he cannot understand if they are explained to him. It does mean that, put on the floor in a safe play room, the baby will exercise according to his needs. If allowed to pull himself up by a crib or chair, he will not stand so long that he will bow his legs. Babies need to climb, to roll, and to bounce, and they deserve a pen or a crib that will give them opportunity to do so.

Some authorities on babyhood discourage the use of baby swings and kiddy-cars — on what grounds it is not known. The baby will bounce, and if the tired or busy mother prefers that he bounce in a safe canvas swing rather than on her lap, she should not be censured. Eventually, too, the baby will use his feet to creep and walk, and what does it matter if a strip of wood and three safe wheels keep him off the floor for brief intervals? Most likely the grounds on which objections to these toys have been made is that they may be used unwisely. The baby may be left in the swing or car till he falls asleep from exhaustion. The wise parent will not put the baby in a swing or car unless he is thoroughly well, rested, and in a playful mood, and then she will not leave him there longer than fifteen or thirty minutes at a time. A half hour of such exercise a day will certainly not harm the healthy baby.

The statement that a baby will not overtax his strength does not rule out the possibility of his being overstimulated to activity. The baby can be romped with until he is nervous and cross, but this is not of his own doing. Fifteen minutes or so of vigorous romping with an adult is enough at one time, and two or three such play periods a day are sufficient. If adults have to be entertained by the baby for longer periods (for in reality the baby is the host and adults are guests at such frolics), they should put the baby on the floor and content themselves with observing his spontaneous antics.

MOTOR PLAY AS AN EXPRESSION OF TREND TOWARD ACTIVITY

Each baby's idiosyncracies in motor development were discussed in some detail in the chapters on walking and individual differences. But it is in his self-initiated play that the baby's joy in activity finds freest expression and by which his true motor ability can best be judged. Outstanding play responses will be tabulated for each baby, and an estimate of his general motor ability will be made.[1]

[1] The total number of Gross Bodily Movement cards is inserted because it gives a rough idea of the amount of motor activity and because it gives a notion of the number of observations upon which the summaries are based. The grammatically unpardonable sequence of tenses in these excerpts from the original records has its purpose. Present tense denotes the development of motor traits that occurred frequently or became habits. Past tense indicates a single occurrence.

Protocols and Summaries

Martin. — Markedly accelerated in motor development. Walking age, 50 weeks. Number of G. B. M. cards (many containing 10 or 12 items), 36.

12 weeks. Lifted trunk when tapeline was pulled under him.

19 weeks. Slid down on B's lap by keeping heels down and lifting buttocks.

24 weeks. Pulls self to standing posture holding B's thumbs, then walks. Begs to do it again and again.

32 weeks. Flopped over on bed and crept away from B during measurement.

34 weeks. Crept and got bell at distance of six feet, then repeatedly threw it ahead and crept after it.

35 weeks. Crept to instrument box and climbed to stand by it; when captured by B he climbed up her.

42 weeks. Pushed examiners' table away with his knee.

47 weeks. Bucks like a broncho in his high chair.

49 weeks. Climbed and walked around box; climbed by fireplace. Crept to stairs and climbed first step three times.

62 weeks. Ran to door, opened it, and escaped into other room. Goes downstairs all alone.

70 weeks. Clings to edge of dresser-top with his fingers and tries to scale up the front to get toys that were put there out of his reach. Almost gets to top of dresser in this way. (Repeats this many times and does it at every succeeding test done in the bedroom and often pulled down a toy by this method.)

78 weeks. Climbed in and out of crib even though the bars were raised to their fullest height.

82 weeks. Ran to kitchen door calling "Papa"; followed mother who had gone to call father to telephone. Takes toys and walks away saying "Bye." Struts around carrying examiners' suitcase of toys.

84 weeks. Climbed up in crib, looked out window, then closed it with one sturdy pull.

86 weeks. Clings to door-knob and scales door. Goes behind

bed, pushes it, then climbs onto iron rail at head of bed and stands looking over arched iron headboard. Stamps and dances over to cedar chest to get picture book. Lifted suitcase of toys off cedar chest, then put it back again, setting it with handle upright, although it was a high reach for him.
90 weeks. Climbs up mother and sits astride her hips. Climbed and stood on cedar chest to reach toys on dresser.
78 weeks and following. Father built a pen in back yard for him, using six-foot chicken wire. When Martin was put into it he immediately climbed to the top. Father had to add an angular guard fence at the top in order to turn him.

Such feats made clear to spectators how myths of babyhood prowess grew up about the names of legendary heroes. Medieval bard might well have sung a lay to Martin's infant strength, his steadfast skill, his staunch, unswerving motor interests. As they watched him charge about the house, slaying such monsters as beset the path of twentieth-century babies, the examiners dubbed him "Infant Hercules." By 6 months he had tamed adults to be his derricks and his steeds; at 8 months he emerged triumphant from his conquest of furniture; and a few weeks later toys went down before his onslaughts.

To Martin activity was no trivial play; it was his life's serious business, the labor in which he reveled. His favorite sport at 7 months was to grasp an adult's thumbs and be swung from bed to floor or jumped or dangled in mid-air. Chairs and tables early bore the imprint of his fingers; beds and sofas yielded to his prancing feet; big motor toys were his delight. During a party given for the babies when they were 10 months old Martin crept away from mother and playmates to tinker with an overturned kiddy-car. At the 2-year-olds' party, where a number of kiddy-cars, trucks, and carts had been lined up for the little guests' use, he straightway made off with an express wagon, the largest toy and one that the other children had completely ignored. At 2 years he was adopting manly standards of chivalry, which in itself is largely motor deference. Eagerly he ran to open doors for mother and stood aside for her to pass; gallantly he escorted the examiners to the steps, carrying their satchel.

His strength and speed of motor development cannot be attributed to his exuberant health. He had a most unpromising start, a breast abscess that put him in the isolation room early in his second week, feeding difficulties arising from the fact that his mother was wholly unable to give him breast milk and that doctors and nurses were unable to discover an adequate formula for him. He remained at the hospital for more than a week after his mother went home. His feeding problems continued, and his mother worried along with a "spitting-up" baby throughout the entire first year, long after other mothers had laid aside bibs and forgotten about them. To the examiners the wonder was that he thrived at all, much less that he became the Samson of the group.

Carol. — Accelerated in motor development. Walking age, 50 weeks. Total number of G. B. M. cards (some containing several items), 11.

35 weeks. Rolled, kicked, gurgled, pounded heels on floor.
46 weeks. Climbed and stood up in high chair between tests.
49 weeks. Sat up three times without help. Climbed by steps and sat down.
62 weeks. Afraid of own shadow; tried to get it by backing up to it.
70 weeks. Walks around during test, scooting on and off B's lap and taking toys to mother.
74 weeks. Joined with brother Ben and S in romping game of hide-and-seek.
78 weeks. Goes to chair and bounces between tests.
104 weeks. Shy; runs to mother repeatedly. Runs to chair where she bounces and hides her face.

Except for her early climbing and walking Carol showed little of the motor play of an accelerated baby. Her motor play was graceful and "ladylike," rather than headlong and boisterous as was that of the precocious boy babies, and for this reason her agile climbing and fleet-footed dancing made less impression on the examiners.

MAXFIELD. — Accelerated in motor development. Walking age, 54 weeks. Total number of G. B. M. cards (to 54 weeks only), 23.

23 weeks. Alternately drew up right and left legs when lying on back as if pedaling a bicycle. Stiffened legs and slid down on B's lap.

34 weeks and following. Climbed in high chair; could not be kept in chair for test.

35 weeks. Crept to get tape. Rollicked and wallowed all over B. Crept to her and climbed on her lap.

43 weeks. Rode well on kiddy-car at party. Charged about all over lawn, leading mother by one finger.

42 to 54 weeks. Creeps and climbs throughout each test; won't sit still to play.

44 weeks. Climbs up steps well; can't come down steps.

50 weeks. Hung to B's neck and shoulders when she sat on floor, trying to get her to take him riding picka-back.

In his early weeks the mother and grandmother of Max expressed anxiety because the baby did not hold up his head and sit alone as did his cousin Rex, who was only 5 days older. The examiners assured the grandmother, who was devoted to both babies, that the performance of Rex was remarkable and that Max, too, was well ahead of other babies in the group. Rex was all but sitting alone at 16 weeks, at which age his parents moved from the city. It is to be regretted that records on him were not available, for he showed promise of being the most precocious baby of the lot.

Maxfield's record was certainly as outstanding as one could wish. He ran close second to Martin in his speed and skill in motor performance. Like Martin and Carol he climbed in his high chair and could not be kept still for a test. His play was almost entirely motor. He raced about the house on his kiddy-car and for months kept his mother and grandmother in leading strings. For more boisterous play his father was his prancing charger, and Max seemed quite nonplused that B did not saddle him on her slender shoulders for a ride about the house.

VIRGINIA RUTH. — Advanced in motor development. Walking age, 54 weeks. Total number of G. B. M. cards, 17.
25 weeks. Plays with toes a great deal.
40 weeks. Rolled off bed; more frightened than hurt.
49 weeks. Walked toward mirror, holding to bed; looked at mirror baby and gurgled. Walks in kiddy-car.
54 weeks. Walked to mirror; toddles alone across floor.
58 to 102 weeks. Frequently walks or runs away during examination.
70 weeks. Strutted around; fell.
72 weeks. Walks upstairs holding to banister; comes down sailing on her stomach.
94 weeks. Put head down in "Mohammedan prayer" posture; fingered toes; acted shy and tried to keep examiners from catching her eye.
102 weeks. Jumped up and down when toys were given. Lay on stomach to play.

Although she was considerably advanced in motor development, Virginia Ruth was certainly the most independent child in showing off her accomplishments. If she were in the mood she rolled, crept, or walked with much enthusiasm; if she were not, neither love, in the form of her mother's coaxing, nor money, in the guise of enticing toys, could induce her to perform. She was an active baby, but, as her mother expressed it, she was a conscientious objector. Her chief objection was at being handled, and even the everyday processes of being dressed and undressed aroused her wrath, which she displayed by screams with vigorous motor accompaniments. When she became able to walk she avoided the distasteful handling by walking out of the situation. She apparently disliked even being watched and sometimes avoided the examiner's scrutiny by absorption in her toes or by an ostrich-like hiding of her head.

Sibyl. — Somewhat advanced in motor development. Walking age, 58 weeks. Total number of G. B. M. cards, 6.
22 weeks. Puts feet up and together.
40 weeks. Walks around garden holding to fence.
42 weeks. Kicks and flops arms when being shown toys.
45 weeks. Hangs over edge of bed and carriage now.
54 weeks. Climbed by bench.
94 weeks. Ran away saying, "Fwaid," when we first came; came back with maid and enjoyed test.
94, 98 weeks. Lay down on stomach to write.

Sibyl was accelerated in her motor development to a slight degree, but her advancement in this phase by no means kept pace with her intellectual precocity. Motor play for its own sake had a minor place in her life; even fine motor coordination and manipulation were not her long suits. Her joy was in examining persons and things, in listening to music, in looking at pictures, in being talked to, and in talking herself. Intellectual pleasure she expressed by motor eagerness, waving and kicking in excitement.

David. — Accelerated in motor development. Walking age, 60 weeks. Total number of G. B. M. cards, 24.
23 weeks. Caught own toes when he could not reach the bell.
30 weeks. Wiggles in high chair; lifted the tray with his feet two times.
37 weeks. Lost interest in toy; crawled to stairs where S sat and tried to climb up first step. Repeatedly crawled away from test.
45 weeks. Pulls little chair and climbs on it to turn light on and off.
54 weeks. Crawled and climbed on davenport; climbed and stood on table. Toddles a few steps.
55 weeks. Tumbled while walking; had a bad bump and was scared; did not walk again till 60 weeks.
66 weeks. Threw ball so hard he fell down.

Strength and precocity were indicated in the early motor play of David. The scarcity of G. B. M. cards after the baby attained walking was due to the fact that he settled down to a good but in no way remarkable standard of motor performance.

JAMES D. — Average in motor development. Walking age, 60 weeks. Total number of G. B. M. cards, 21.
19 weeks. Noticed feet for first time.
24 weeks. Caught toes; transferred hand from right to left toes when B transferred from left to right foot in measuring.
37 weeks. Shudders and grimaces from excitement.
48 weeks. Beginning to use kiddy-car; at first he could only go backward but now travels nicely.
48 weeks. Becomes very excited and happy when undressed for bath and will crawl toward bathroom when undressed if he is put on the floor and "bath" is mentioned to him.
50 weeks. Stands in high chair and rocks it back and forth.
66 weeks. Walked to door to meet examiners.
74 weeks. Drummed heels on floor while waiting for B to bring toys.
86 weeks. Ran off to 38th Street (one-half block away across a through-traffic street).

Jimmy's motor play was about as typical as that of any baby for illustrating the motor trend at different levels. He took an average amount of exercise in an ordinary way, but motor play was not one of his chief delights or modes of expression.

HARVEY. — Average in motor development. Walking age, 62 weeks. Total number of G. B. M. cards, 53.
26 weeks. Plays "Draw a bucket of water for the farmer's daughter" with mother. When game is over mother says "Shall we play it again?" Baby swings and pulls mother's arm to signify his desire to do so.
32, 33, 39 weeks. Bounces in buggy, bed, and swing; at mother's command "Bouncie, bouncie" he begins to bounce in swing.
22, 33 to 40 weeks. Plays with toes a great deal; kicks and scrubs heels together; sits watching his moving feet.

44 weeks. Rides kiddy-car; shouts for help when he is stuck.
47 weeks. Wants to stand up when riding in carriage.
54, 55 weeks. Kiddy-car polo is his favorite game; he rides around kicking a ball all over the floor.
64 weeks. Plays hide-and-seek, running after older brother when he hides.
78 weeks. Climbs on davenport and chairs but will not climb off. Calls for mother and as soon as she appears starts walking off even though she is not near enough to reach him.
78 weeks. Coyly put head down on floor, peeked at B, and when she looked at him put his head down again; looked at S, started to put head down as if shy, looked at her again to be sure that she was watching him, and since she appeared not to, did not continue his coy hiding. Repeated the same trick with B two times.
94 weeks. Backed up, creeping on the floor, scooted away, looked back and smiled; peeked through back of chair; pushed chair with feet, looked around, and smiled, bidding for attention. Performed monkeyshines and wanted to show off as long as anyone would watch him.
98 weeks. Walked about, swaggering; lay flat on floor and kicked toes.
98 weeks. Discovered that light globes pop when they are dropped; now goes around, climbs on chairs, unscrews bulbs, and throws them to make them pop.

The early motor play of Harvey gave expression to his general personality trend of slashing, kicking, and patting. During his second year he, too, staged clever and daring stunts, but unlike those of Don his acts always seemed to be done with eyes on the gallery. He wanted attention, and he used his best stunts and his most winning smiles to get it.

WINIFRED. — Average or accelerated in motor development. Walking age, 62 weeks. Total number of G. B. M. cards, 11.
15 weeks. Sat on bed, propped with pillows, facing her twin, Fred. Leaned toward him.
21 to 26 weeks. Vigorously jumps in baby swing.

40 weeks. Stood in carriage and fell out; not seriously hurt.
68 weeks. Carried chair to davenport and thus climbed on it.
78 weeks. Runs errands, taking soiled clothes to hamper, etc.
98 weeks. Dramatized "Little Jack Horner" when mother said the rhyme.

WILLIAM FREDERICK. — Slow in motor development. Walking age, 70 weeks. Total number of G. B. M. cards, 14.
18 weeks. Jounced up and down, waving arms and kicking when daddy and brothers scuffled.
21 to 26 weeks. Enjoys baby swing.
33 weeks. Kicks with excitement when cap and sweater are put on.
78 weeks. Helps run errands with sister.
82 weeks. Trots after B to get more toys. Climbs in and out of own chair.
98 weeks. Pushed down 8-block tower, then fell himself to illustrate its downfall. Dramatized "Jack and Jill" and "Humpty Dumpty" for mother by falling at proper words.

The play of these twins contained relatively little of gross motor elements, especially of the play-for-exercise's-sake type. From the outset Winifred surpassed Fred in both skill and speed in activity; indeed, according to the mother's report the difference existed before birth, for Winifred was a vigorous prenatal kicker whereas Fred was quiet.[2] Movies of the twins at 40 weeks showed Winifred standing beside a toy auto, while Fred sat watching, pat-a-caking, and shaking his head and saying, "No-No." Fred compensated for his lack of motor skill by jabbering. So marked were these motor and vocal differences between the twins at 10 months that older children in the family nicknamed the pair "Winnie Walker" and "Freddie Talker." (See Plate 6, page 71.)

In their later development these babies showed a tendency to act with a purpose and to make each movement count. They easily attached meaning to their motor play, acquired

[2] The physician's report of the prenatal position of each baby and the order of birth of the twins enabled the mother to identify the little kicker.

a sense of the dramatic and a good notion of how to express themselves. Capable and systematic training on the part of the mother did much to direct the activities of the twins into interesting and helpful outlets.

QUENTIN. — Average in motor development. Walking age, 64 weeks. Total G. B. M. cards, 15.
37 weeks. Raises chair tray above head with feet.
41 weeks. Stood in crib, took stockings and blanket off rail, tried to replace them, and succeeded with stockings.
45 weeks. Watched B put bell on chair; went creeping for it with a whoop.
48 weeks. Stands playing on piano.
54 weeks. Climbed and put handkerchief on smoking stand.
66 weeks. Walks on knees like a "penitent sinner" as his mother says.
98 weeks. Sits clapping feet together while waiting for B to get toys.

This baby's motor development proceeded at the average rate; he devoted only a moderate part of his time to motor pursuits but took great delight in them. Like Larry he was content to sit playing quietly with manipulative toys for hours at a time. Although he enjoyed the tests and was eager for each new toy to be brought, he did not leap to his feet and scamper after the examiner but sat with nervous patience waiting till the next toy was brought.

MAURICE. — Average in motor development. Walking age, 66 weeks. Total number of G. B. M. cards (many containing several items), 19.
5 weeks. At bath tried to get to his feet.
38 weeks. Sits playing with his toes.
48 weeks. Propels kiddy-car a little but doesn't seem to enjoy it unless someone is with him.
49 weeks. Leaned over and bit top of box that lay on floor, pulled lid off with teeth, and pushed box on floor with nose.
54 to 102 weeks. Repeatedly creeps or runs away during ex-

amination; sometimes escapes with toy; has a regular circuit, living room, dining room, hall, kitchen, dining room, living room. Examinations become a game of "follow-the-leader," with Maurice the leader and B and S the followers. Also climbs on chairs and runs to doors. Won't sit still to look at pictures, though he sometimes can be corralled for manipulative tests.

88 weeks. In walking test, B started to lead him but he fussed and pulled back and went for oil bottle that he usually carries to S when he walks down path to her, but this time B left bottle on floor. Mother put him back on paper but his walking was not typical.

90 weeks. Leaned over and kissed paper that was put on floor for him to write on.

Just as Maurice held certain traits of temperament in common with Matthew and Virginia Ruth, so he approximated them in motor play. In common with them he was easily provoked to lusty crying. During the first year he was frequently incensed by the manipulation involved in being measured, and his play, too, was independent. He had the escape motive very strongly and delighted in walking out on the examiners. Like them he had mannerisms indicating an unwillingness to be spied upon in his play; bowing to the floor to nose along a toy was a way of paying elaborate inattention to the examiners. Very similar reactions were reported for Virginia Ruth.

JUDY.—Average in walking development. Walking age, 66 weeks. Total number of G. B. M. cards, 20.

35 weeks. Pats hands on thighs, waves, and gurgles in excitement.

41 weeks. Sings and dances by shaking body when told to sing and dance. Bounces, jumps, and jiggles.

58 weeks. Climbed and stood by examiner's box, then sat down backward.

66, 74, 78, 86, 90 weeks. Wanted more toys; between each test got up and trotted to buffet and pointed for next toy.

74 weeks. Scrambled on davenport and seated herself between mother and S; slid off and went to see what toy B was bringing her.
74 to 104 weeks. Usually runs down paper to S with arms outspread and laughing.
94 weeks. Judy was taken to train to meet mother who was returning from a long trip. When she saw her mother Judy stiffened out and cried "Muddie" about ten times and ran to meet her.

In motor play Judy showed few peculiarities. She was active and playful, but motor play was not her chief delight. She resembled Don and Sibyl in her kicking and waving in anticipation and pleasure. Like Torey she was very social and friendly, and hence most of her motor wants were supplied for her. Vocalization was a great outlet for her energies as it was for William Frederick.

Irene May. — Somewhat slow in motor development. Walking age, 66 weeks. Total number of G. B. M. cards (records to 76 weeks only), 6.
21, 22 weeks. Lifts body from toe to head when lying on back.
40 weeks. Shakes crib and carriage. Stands in crib and tries to stand in carriage.
68 weeks. Was playing with father, chasing him around the dining-room table. When he got a bit more than halfway round ahead of her she whirled and went the other direction, apparently seeing that the distance was shorter.

Renie May's lack of skill and interest in gross motor pursuits is indicated by the small number of notes on motor behavior. Although her records stopped at 76 weeks, there were few gaps in her records until that time, and her mother kept very complete daily accounts. Most of the time the baby played quietly on the floor, manipulating her dolls and other small toys.

Peter. — Somewhat slow in motor development. Walking age, 66 weeks. Total number of G. B. M. cards, 5.
32 weeks. Sat stolidly looking around.

49 weeks. Abandoned toy for creeping to radio where his twin, Patty, sat. Climbed to knees by radio. Patty crawled away.
70 weeks. Took ball and walked into farthest corner of room. No interest in playing with B.
107 weeks. Played with shoes.

PATRICIA. — Somewhat slow in motor development. Walking age, 70 weeks. Total number of G. B. M. cards, 12.
20 weeks. Arches back so that trunk is off table; kicks heels on table, thus progressing backward.
54 weeks. Scrambled onto B's lap, climbed by chair.
70 weeks. After the walking test held oil bottle and rubbed toes as if oiling them.
79 weeks. Stood and put head down as if for a somersault.
54 to 107 weeks. Frequently climbed up on B's lap to sit for test; often put her arm around B. Liked to cuddle.

Peter and Patricia were not interested in taking exercise. "They are such lazy babies," was their mother's frequent comment, and indeed they were. They sat on the floor playing with whatever was within arm's reach and were contented just to sit in their carriage sunning themselves and watching passers-by. They were very social babies and greatly enjoyed being held and cuddled.

WALLEY. — Slow in motor development. Walking age, 68 weeks. Total number of G. B. M. cards, 12.
4 weeks. Lifted trunk when tape was slipped under.
35 weeks. Bounces on floor and bed.
49 weeks. Crept to our box, scrambled across B's legs, and climbed to knees by davenport.
66 weeks. Got up during test and walked to window to see milk wagon.
78 weeks. Drummed heels.

Walley's play was of the eager but inactive sort. He often struggled to get toys that were out of his range and did the usual amount of creeping and climbing, but like Fred and Renie May he spared himself motor activity and depended on adults to do for him the things his own legs could not do.

DONOVAN. — Slow in motor development. Walking age, 70 weeks. Total number of G. B. M. cards (some containing several items), 46.
16 weeks. Steps with left foot so that he goes round in a circle.
20 to 40 weeks. Goes after toes; whets toes together; puts soles of feet together.
28 to 50 weeks. Kicks and bounces eagerly when he wants someone to get him or when asked if he wants to go "bye-bye." Bounces in car and in carriage, in fact is always jumping when he is awake. Bounces if he likes a thing and to express excitement.
34 weeks. Doesn't do the things he used to do such as rolling and pulling self up, because he is weak from illness.
40 weeks. Jumps and yells at parents to scare them.
51 weeks. Sometimes rolls around when sitting up.
62 weeks. Sat under table and held bottle in both hands above his head, looked at it, then leaned forward and put it down on floor, lifted, and repeated, bowing like Oriental dancer using incense bowl at worship. Jabbers in sentences throughout this performance.
74 weeks. Walks away with toy, swaggering and strutting.
78, 82, 90, 104 weeks. Lies down on stomach to look at picture book, evidently imitating his brother's favorite reading posture.
86 weeks. Gets up in middle of test and runs to window to look out; comes back dancing.
90 weeks. Sits crossing and uncrossing legs.
104 weeks. Imitates mother's and Examiner B's standing postures.

Although Don's motor performance was not in the least precocious it was strikingly individualistic and histrionic. Of all babies Don was the most ardently interested in playing with his toes and the most eager bouncer. His delight in mimicry and buffoonery began to show up in his ninth and tenth months. His comedy was not for the sake of attracting an audience; for him it was spontaneous fun. To be sure, he enjoyed the attention it brought him. Not even the matter-of-fact scientific observers, much less doting parents and a 12-year-old brother comedian, could fail to stop work when this baby chose to favor them with an act. Like an actor sure of his audience and confident of his talents Don serenely did his number and then looked up for the applause he expected as his due and knew was forthcoming. He, too, compensated for late walking by a great deal of jabbering. Repeatedly his mother described him as a "great talker" and S had difficulty in describing his antics and recording his speech at the same time.

Torey. — Very slow in walking. Walking age, 74 weeks. Total number of G. B. M. cards, 12.
18 weeks. Held to sides of tub and pulled self upward.
29 weeks. Seated, leaned forward, and put toe of shoe in mouth.
35 weeks. Bounces back and forth on floor.
45 to 50 weeks. Creeps and climbs. Drops toys especially to stand on B's lap so he can look at her face and converse with her.
68 weeks. Mother reported that before he had the flu two weeks ago he had walked a great deal led by only one hand; has not walked much since, although he will walk when mother leads him. Sat down; made no effort at walking test. Would not climb to standing position by furniture although he formerly did so.
74 weeks. Climbed and put bell on davenport. Walks by himself.

Torey was a baby whose early motor development proceeded at the normal rate. When it came to managing his legs for walking, however, he met with difficulties. His very tiny, short feet and short legs and his round, heavy trunk seemed to make the assumption of an upright posture very hard for him, and illness at a crucial age probably accentuated his retardation. Sociability was his trump card, and not until winning smiles and bidding calls had failed to give him the attention of adults did he resort to motor play.

Larry. — Very slow in walking. Walking age, 76 weeks. Total number of G. B. M. cards, 16.

30 weeks. Arms outspread; pounces on objects eagerly.
35 weeks. Shakes head, dips head and looks up under brows, and acts smart.
51 weeks. Has invented a game of putting pillow behind shoulders and throwing it forward over head. Hitches about following older children as they run about the house. Squeals and jabbers as he goes.
66 weeks. Sways shoulders and head to jazz music.
78 weeks. Came to door with grandmother to greet examiners.
98 weeks. Can come downstairs alone now. Climbed on chair at end of examination and called "Mammee" to look at him.

Gross motor performance had little place in Larry's play. He was clever at manipulation and at fine motor skill but for a long time made no attempts at moving himself.

MATTHEW. — Accelerated in motor development. No record of walking age. Total number of G. B. M. cards, 22. (Records on this baby were incomplete because he was older than the others, and his tests were preliminary and experimental.)
13 weeks. Mother found him biting toe.
16 weeks. Lifted trunk when tapeline was put under; clasped legs around examiner's arm.
33 weeks. Shook head hard and fast.
45 weeks. Throws toys in front; creeps after them.
49 weeks. Crawled to door and closed it; it required three pushes.
49 weeks. Bounces and gurgles when dog or cat is near; tries to catch it.
51 weeks. Climbed one stair step, pulled telephone, which was on landing, over on his head; hasn't tried to climb since.
74 weeks. Climbed on examiner's box and stood upright on it.
74 weeks. Crawls upstairs and down.
86, 90, and 98 weeks. Had temper tantrums; rolled on floor, kicked, and screamed.
74 to 102 weeks. Repeatedly walked or ran off at examinations, often taking toy along or going to hunt examiners' instrument box,which intrigued him greatly.

If his records had been more complete, the motor development of Matthew probably would have ranked alongside that of Max in precocity. His motor play was always skillful and strenuous. At a very early age he began to use vigorous kicking and slashing as a defense against the confinement of being dressed or measured. Later he exhibited temper tantrums accompanied by all the motor adjuncts.

Doris. — Early acceleration. Total G. B. M. cards before 60 weeks, 22.

19 weeks. Tries to talk to brother, raising herself to half-sitting posture in bed.

23 weeks. "Rock-a-byes" on mother's lap at her command.

32 weeks. Tries to dance like her daddy when she hears music. Rolls over in bath when mother tells her to.

38 weeks. Plays peeka-boo, rolling on stomach to hide her face.

49 weeks. Crawls over for someone to pity her if she is hurt.

No baby exceeded Doris in precision and grace of movement. Her early skill at walking and her quick learning of motor tricks forecast for her a splendid motor career. She often assumed statuesque poses, arching her lithe, slender body in the perfect form of a dancer or diver. Her early death marked a loss to science as well as to her devoted family.

Summary

In the baby's motor play two factors seem to be operating, first, the factor of the pattern of motor development, which makes him play up to but not beyond the limits of his particular stage of development, and, second, the factor of individuality, which makes him play according to the dictates of his own physical strength and his interest in activity. The former makes for similarity in the quality of motor play of different babies at the same developmental level; the latter makes for differences among them in quantity of motor play and in the ends toward which their play is directed. The first should make for consistency between motor play and physical development and to a lesser degree between motor play and the level of intellectual performance. The second should make motor play a consistent expression of personality traits. Babies having similar personality traits should therefore have similar play interests, or vice versa.

Since individual summaries are hard to compare, perhaps one may be forgiven for recapitulating. Matthew, Maurice, and Virginia Ruth had in common the traits of irritability at being handled and general motor independence. This personality trait was often expressed in the motor accompaniments of tantrums in the early weeks and by walking away from the examination as soon as locomotion was possible. Fred, Don, and Walley, who were large, comfortable, good-natured babies but slow in motor development, had motor expressions of eagerness to be picked up and carried about, and all made up for clumsy feet by glib tongues. Martin and Max were strong and strenuous and were never so happy as when exercising. Carol, Sibyl, Winifred, and James were proficient enough at motor play, but they took exercise in moderation and more for the sake of than to the exclusion of social and intellectual pursuits.

There is no need to amplify the argument by further examples; it is enough to say that each baby plays in accordance with his motor abilities and his personal interests. Parents need not worry that their baby may wear himself out at bouncing or standing or that they may fail to give him practice in walking at the crucial moment. If the baby has the urge to bounce or stand, he will find a way to do so, and if he is not yet ready to walk, the most patient of parents will find their practice exercises in vain.

CHAPTER XI

THEORETICAL IMPLICATIONS OF LOCOMOTOR DEVELOPMENT

If orderliness of motor pattern and individuality of motor interests are the two outstanding factors in locomotor development, how are they to be accounted for? The assembled data furnish no direct evidence as to the causes of either phenomenon, but they point toward the conclusions that the one is a function of maturation and the other corresponds to a talent.

EVIDENCE FAVORING THE MATURATION HYPOTHESIS

Maturation has long been a moot point in genetic psychology. Woodworth (40) has strongly advanced the notion that walking development is a process of maturation rather than of learning, but he gives only anecdotal evidence in support of his statements. Observation and experiment on habits have convinced Watson, Sherman, and Gesell on the theory of maturation, the former two as to its falsity, the latter as to its truth.

With regard to the point Watson (38)[1] puts into the mouth of the modern mother the question, "Isn't it just possible that almost nothing is given by heredity and that practically the whole course of development of the child is due to the way I raise it?" He further queries, "Aren't such activities as climbing, imitation . . . play . . . shyness . . . pure instincts which appear and run their course completely beyond the control of parents?" and replies:

[1] *Psychological Care of Infant and Child*, pp. 37, 38.

The behaviorist believed, when he began work, that some of these acts would spring forth fully formed. But we waited for their appearance in vain. Now we are forced to believe from the study of facts that all of these forms of behavior are *built in* by the parent and by the environment which the parent allows the child to grow up in.

With regard to motor development in particular he says:

Other activities appear at a later stage — such as blinking, reaching, handling, handedness, crawling, standing, sitting up, walking, running, jumping. *In the great majority of these later activities it is difficult to say how much of the act as a whole is due to training and conditioning. A considerable part is unquestionably due to the growth changes in structure, and the remainder is due to training and conditioning.*

Sherman (27)[2] speaks in like vein:

The first overt bodily reactions of the newborn infant are simple sensori-motor responses which are strikingly undefined, uncoordinated, and aimless. With the increase in age and experience these reactions of the bodily musculature become guided and usefully coordinated, indicating that most of the complex behavior of the growing infant is the result of a direct learning activity rather than the manifestation of inherited modes of response.

In favor of maturation Gesell (13) maintains that infant behavior follows a pattern that depends upon intrinsic physiological conditions, and "that the physiological process of maturation determines in a large measure the form and sequence of infant behavior pattern" just as certainly as the hydrogen-ion concentration of the blood directs and controls respiration. He deplores the lack of work on this important point and advocates his method of comparing the performance of an untrained twin with that of his trained identical twin

[2] *The Process of Human Behavior*, p. 61.

as a way of making crucial tests of the maturation hypothesis.

But crucial tests of maturation on the entire course of motor development and on a large number of identical twins will probably never be made. So long as the shadow of a doubt about the changeless onsweep of development crosses the psychologist's mind, so long will he hesitate to perform crucial tests. He will not chance the atrophy of the walking process of one baby by keeping him cooped in a pen where use of his limbs would be impossible; nor will he risk endangering the physique of a twin by putting him through a stiff set of paces in the hope of speeding up his motor development. And even if the psychologist himself were persuaded that he would hazard the future of neither twin, few parents would give him free rein with their babies. Gesell himself intimates that the stair-climbing experiment that promised so much for the co-twin control method was made possible largely by the death of the twins' mother, after which the babies became accessible for daily training in his institute. In view of the certain difficulties and possible dangers of crucial experiments it is up to the psychologist to glean all possible evidence on maturation from observations of development as it proceeds in its usual way.

Deducing the Course of Motor Development from the Maturation Hypothesis

Granting for the moment the truth of the maturation hypothesis, let us consider the general nature and special features of motor development as they would take place with maturation at the helm. In what way does maturation proceed, and how would its course affect motor development?

Maturation an orderly course. — All physical growth, as far as we know, takes place in an orderly manner. The child does not reach a height of 3 feet without at some time having been 2 feet 6 inches tall; the caterpillar does not become a butterfly without first having been a pupa. So it would seem that motor development, guided by maturation, should steer an orderly course, each stage being the natural outcome of the one going before and the prerequisite for the one coming after.

Course unaltered by speed of development. — That growth proceeds at different rates in different individuals is a truism. But the course of normal development shows little mutability. The development of the frog's egg can be accelerated by the use of thyroxin. Nevertheless, the order of development is still embryo, tadpole, frog; the tadpole stage is never skipped. By analogy, the maturation of walking should proceed by stages that are neither omitted nor reversed in order.

Sudden appearance of maturing functions. — Experiments on animals seem to indicate that a trait depending on maturation may show itself suddenly, and observations on humans lead to the same conclusion. The hair of a baby's chin does not lengthen and coarsen gradually until in early manhood he has a beard. Instead, the boy's face is smooth until puberty, and then within a few months the beard is grown. One might expect similar abrupt transitions from stage to stage in motor development.

Maturation an anatomical and physiological process. — Growth is a physiological process that takes place in time and space. The time element is probably the one that differentiates maturing functions such as the attainment of height from nonmaturing functions such as breathing and digestion. If motor development is a maturing function, it, too, should be strongly dependent upon the time or age element, and it should have physiological or anatomical correlates age by age. Motor development, if dependent on maturation, should proceed in harmony with the laws of physiological maturation.

Other Hypotheses That Might Account for Motor Development

Before testing the facts of motor development for conformity with the above requirements it is well to consider on what bases other than maturation the pattern of motor development might be explained. Three other hypotheses suggest themselves: first, that motor sequence is a function of learning; second, that it is wholly dependent on chance; and third, that it can be attributed to a combination of the three, maturation, learning, and chance.

The learning theory. — By learning is meant the slow and toilsome process whereby ground is gained by practice. Accepting the learning hypothesis as the sole explanation of motor development would lead to the following consequences:

1. Individual differences in motor development would agree with differences in amount of practice and with opportunities and training that parents give the babies.

2. There would be little or no orderliness in motor development. By pure trial and error learning some babies would certainly hit upon a method of walking before they crept or of creeping before they sat alone. With the parents, moreover, walking is the goal toward which training is directed. They do not put the baby through a course of swimming movements in order to teach him

to walk. Difference in training methods between parents would undoubtedly make for differences in motor sequence in babies, provided parental training was effective.

3. Furthermore, the random efforts of the baby or the directed efforts of his parents would lead the baby to skip one or more stages of development. Mothers would surely train the baby to skip the creeping stage if they could and would curb the climbing stage. Babies themselves might prefer to omit the content-to-sit-in-a-high-chair stage.

4. Finally, the onset of each stage of learning development would be gradual rather than sudden; daily practice would result in noticeable daily improvement or at least in noticeable weekly improvement.

The chance theory. — If chance alone dictated the course of motor development, consistency in sequence between babies would be the exception rather than the rule. Five motor stages completely permutable could stand in 120 different orders, and if 5 stages leading to creeping were completely permutable with 5 stages leading to sitting alone and 5 others leading to walking, the possible orders of development would be a factorial 15, or 872,183,012,000. Even partial permutability would lead to astoundingly large numbers of possible orders.

The combination theory. — A combination of the three factors would seem on the surface to be the most tenable of the three theories. If, however, chance entered into the developmental order at all it would lead to great permutability and hence to a chaotic sequence, and if learning played a significant rôle it would lead to gradual development and to a tendency to skip stages in the sequence.

Testing the Maturation Hypothesis

Motor development orderly. — The orderly unfolding of motor development has been stressed in the preceding chapters. Motor development follows a pattern.[3] The five stages of the general pattern have been termed for the sake of convenience, passive postural control of upper trunk, active postural control of entire trunk, effort toward locomotion, locomotion by creeping, and walking alone. Some may say that these five stages are so general and so simple that they can hardly be called stages at all and that this order is just what one would expect. But there is orderliness in the development of a particular motor skill; creeping, sitting, and standing all have their patterns. Because it follows a pattern, motor development meets the requirements of the maturation hypothesis.

Pattern consistent regardless of speed. — The point has already been made that all babies go through the same stages of development in approximately the same sequence even though for some babies a given stage may be long and for others, short. Speed of motor development is an individual characteristic, just as is rate of physical growth. Since differences in speed of motor development apparently bear no relation to the parents' efforts to train the babies, and since orderliness of developmental sequence persists in spite of differences in speed, the learning theory is considerably shaken. The fact that speed does not alter the sequence of motor development is another confirmation of the maturation hypothesis.

[3] The term "pattern" has brewed much palaver and little research among psychologists and has long served as a cloak for ignorance. The author uses the word here to mean a demonstrable arrangement of reactions in a time sequence, the existence of which has been established through long continued

Suddenness of new phases of motor development.—Some may criticize the presentation of these data in stages or orders on the ground that such terms endow motor development with a hitch-and-halt aspect that it does not really possess. On the contrary, motor development, if it be a true analogy of physical growth, should proceed by gradual increments. A criticism of this sort can be met only by admitting that the terms "stage" and "order" do give such an impression, but a step-by-step presentation of the material pictures motor development with far greater fidelity to the observed facts than does any term implying that motor development proceeds by gradual daily or weekly increments. All the babies seemed to improve by spurts. For weeks at a time a child remained at a standstill and suddenly within a day's time he had climbed the next step and was functioning on an entirely different motor level. To be sure, there was some noticeable improvement in sitting, creeping, or walking for a few days after the reaction was established, but creeping certainly did not keep on improving until walking began, nor did the ability to stand and walk by holding to furniture blend imperceptibly into the ability to walk alone.

The transition from creeping to walking alone usually came suddenly according to the mothers' reports. Certainly it often happened that a baby who plumped himself down on the floor the moment he was left standing alone for the one-minute test trotted about the house with great unconcern a fortnight later. At one examination the mother expressed fear that her baby might never walk; at the next she despaired at his proclivity for running around and getting into mischief.

observation rather than postulated from logical analysis of the function in question.

"I must tell you," said James Dalton's mother, "Jimmy walked well the night after you last measured him. Just before dinner I ran to the corner grocery on an errand. When I came back there walked Jimmy to the door to meet me! And he walked the whole evening long. After dinner his daddy and I sat and watched him pace up and down and up and down this room. He must have made fifty trips if he made one. We laughed until we cried at the little fellow's perseverance."

Torey's mother for weeks had been alarmed at her son's slowness in walking. When at 74 weeks the boy trotted to the door to greet the experimenters, they exclaimed, "So Torey finally walked." "Finally walked!" his mother replied. "He certainly did. He began last Thursday and he has hardly stopped since."

Winifred's father is authority for an interesting description of the little girl's first efforts to walk. "Winnie discovered she could walk the other night. She got to a standing position in the middle of the floor and took about three steps alone. She wasn't very sure of her balance, so she crawled away to an open space where there was nothing to bother her and there she stood up and sat down, stood again and sat. She practiced for almost an hour. She's walking well now."

Some babies seemed to develop much more suddenly than others. With Larry and Edith Ann it seemed to be characteristic never to attempt a new skill until it could be done to perfection. Time after time with all of the babies the examiners noted a new phase with surprise. No previous observation had led them to suspect that a turn in events was about to take place. Suddenness in development is in accord with the maturation theory.

The above statement must not be interpreted to mean that maturation itself goes on by fits and starts. The maturation that leads to motor development is a matter of bone and muscle growth, increase in the leg-trunk ratio, decrease in the weight-height ratio, and possibly a shift in the center of gravity. Such growth takes place gradually. But motor development waits on muscle growth; when all these anatomical features have reached a minimum development a new motor phase may spring forth. The progress that takes place between one motor stage and the next in terms of muscle growth and neuro-muscular organization is often imperceptible in terms of motor function.

Suddenness of appearance is a characteristic common to the acquisition of all gross motor skills. The boy who "learns" to ride a bicycle makes little or no progress at first, and the advice of his elders to "turn your front wheel the other way if you are about to fall" helps him very little. After repeated starts and falls the boy one day achieves balance and rides off; thereafter he has no trouble, for his knowledge of bicycle-riding is neuro-muscular rather than verbal. Similarly the adult "gets the hang" of a new dance step after a few awkward attempts. Such motor activities are commonly considered to be learned reactions. But like the baby's walking they do not show the gradual increase that comes about from long and patient practice. Suddenness of motor learning is like the solution of a problem by insight, and yet one cannot attribute insight to nerves and muscles.

An "all-or-none" law of motor activity. — Perhaps the reason motor skills partake more largely of an "all-or-none" rather than of a "more-or-less" character is that neuro-muscular coordination obeys an all-or-none law.

If all the nerves and muscles involved in a motor performance act together as they should, the act is perfect, and if any one nerve or muscle fails to cooperate the act is impossible. Is it not logical that the all-or-none law, which has been demonstrated to hold for both nervous conduction and muscle contraction, should hold equally well for complex motor acts, which are possible only by the harmonious working together of many muscles that are enervated by many nerve impulses?

Since walking and bicycle-riding are alike in that both develop suddenly, why cannot both be attributed to maturation? The conclusion probably is not as absurd as it sounds. Once maturation is sufficient there is nothing to hinder the baby from perfecting his neuromuscular coordination or from getting the knack of walking. All his equipment is ready for use, and he need not wait on ceremony. With the boy bicycle-rider, however, one more thing is necessary, a bicycle, and there is little chance of his getting a bicycle just at the moment he is physically mature enough to use one. If babies were naturally endowed with bicycles at birth, it is not at all unlikely that bicycle-riding would be easily recognized to be as maturing a function as walking.

Anatomical correlates of motor development.—Like other maturing functions motor development is strongly dependent upon the time or age factor. Anatomical correlates of motor development have already been discussed at length. Perhaps the most striking example of orderliness in motor development corresponding to orderliness in anatomical development is to be seen in the cephelad-to-caudad progress toward assuming an upright posture.

CONCLUSIONS

All requirements deduced from the maturation hypothesis are met by the data in the following three ways: Motor development proceeds in an orderly sequence regardless of speed of development; new stages often appear suddenly, a fact that suggests that a motor skill is an all-or-none process of coordination dependent upon complete maturation; and motor development has its correlates in physical development. Arguments favoring the learning or the chance theories are badly crippled by the orderly sequence of motor stages. If learning does occur in motor development it takes place through practicing the elements of the act and not through practicing the act itself. A coordinated motor act appears suddenly; it is not the culmination of a patient piling up of small motor increments. In the light of these data the maturation hypothesis is certainly the most tenable of the three theories.

EVIDENCE FAVORING THE TALENT HYPOTHESIS

The maturation theory still leaves unaccounted for the large individual differences in motor development and motor interests. For ages people have known that certain traits run in families. Animal breeders have never questioned that traits can be bred in or out of stock. A predisposition or talent for music or art has long been postulated to account for differences between genius and mediocrity in those lines, and mechanical skill has recently been looked upon as a natural gift rather than as the product of training alone. Is it not possible that a tendency to good motor coordination is a talent also? Great athletes might ascribe their prowess to long years of systematic training, but a good jockey would never train a draft horse for racing.

Deducing the Nature of Differences in Motor Development from the Talent Hypothesis

As in the case of the maturation hypothesis let us picture the nature of motor differences as they would be displayed if the talent hypothesis were true and then examine the data for their conformity to the requirements of the hypothesis.

1. Motor talent would lead to great differences in speed of motor development.

2. Motor talent would be revealed by differences in motor skill.

3. Differences in speed of development and in skill would appear independent of training.

4. These differences would persist over a long period of time.

5. Motor talent or lack of it would have its spontaneous expression in motor play and would fit in with other personality manifestations.

Testing the Data for Conformity to the Hypothesis

Differences in speed of development. — The wide distribution in the age of developing motor functions has been emphasized in Chapter VII. A range of 4 to 8 weeks was necessary to include the ages of the middle 50 per cent of the group in the development of postural control, sitting, creeping, and walking. The entire range in walking age was no less than 6 months. This fulfills the first requirement of the talent hypothesis.

Differences in motor skill. — As has been stated, no measures of difference in motor skill were made because no quantitative scoring method could be devised, but the examiners had a definite impression that great differences in skill existed. Awkward, clumsy, toddling, ponderous, and unsteady are words that well describe the activity of some babies; light on the feet, nimble, sure-footed, sprightly, graceful, and staunch describe that of others. If a measuring scale had been applied it is likely that data would have confirmed descriptions.

Differences appearing without training. — No estimate can be made either of the baby's spontaneous practice or of the parents' efforts to train him. Again the observers had to rely upon their impression that the baby's spontaneous practice was governed by his interest and delight in motor play and that these factors set standards for the type of training in romping and play given by parents. One or two mothers mentioned that they "practiced the baby" for the walking test, but the observers could detect no startling improvement on the baby's part.

Differences in motor activity appeared too early to be ascribable to practice. Indeed, the differences between Winnie and Fred were first observed by the mother during pregnancy. Subsequent differences in their development can hardly be attributed to training or even to early conditioning.

Let it be said here that the early conditioning argument is very hard to refute. Conditioning, so its upholders would have us believe, may come about through a single vivid experience. Who can watch or shield a baby so closely that in the course of three months he will have not a single vivid experience, and who can know what experience is vivid enough to the baby to condition him and what experience is not? The belief that a baby inherits only his reflexes and gets all his emotional and personality traits through conditioning leaves just as impassable a gulf in our knowledge as does belief that he gets them from his grandfather through the medium of a gene. Training and conditioning unquestionably play a rôle in motor development, but their rôle is subservient to maturation and inborn trends.

Persistence of motor trends. — Differences in speed of motor development and more important differences in motor interest and activity did persist over a two-year period. How much longer they will persist cannot be predicted. The author has such faith in their persistence over a long period that could a foot race, a tree-climbing contest, or a long hike be scheduled today to take place ten years hence, the participants to include only the boys of this group, granting there had been no devastating illnesses during the interval and that training had been entirely spontaneous, she would stake odds on a winner.

Spontaneous expression in motor play. — The characteristic ways in which the babies exercise themselves have been dealt with in the preceding chapter. Here again the possibility that training or conditioning dictated the channels of activity cannot be denied, but the probability that differences in play may be accounted for on that basis are slight. It is inconceivable that parents would train their baby to scale the front of a chiffonier or to climb to the top of a 6-foot fence. Rather they would condition him against those things if they could. To be sure, the baby learned or was trained to ride on an adult's shoulder, but parents surely would not have persisted in such play if the baby had not liked it. One mother wrote on the mother's blank in answer to "How does the baby react to being tossed in the air?" "We don't do it any more because the baby doesn't like it. She cries." The fifth requirement seems to be met; the talent hypothesis is satisfied.

Summary

The hypothesis that motor skill corresponds to a talent is supported by evidence, but what the nature of motor talent might be is a matter for speculation. Chief among its components seems to be a neuro-muscular tendency toward good gross motor coordination. It is just as logical that such a tendency can be transmitted through a gene as that the tendencies toward fine motor coordination that make one person an artist and another a pianist are inherited. But there is something more than a tendency toward good coordination; there is an interest in motor pursuits, which is a component of the talent.

Perhaps it seems from the stress put on the maturation and talent theories that the importance of training has been overlooked. It has not. Spontaneous practice is considered only as a manifestation of an urge to motor activity, which arises partly from the maturation of neuro-muscular systems and partly from an inborn predisposition to activity. Motor training imposed upon the baby can be effective only within limits that are circumscribed by anatomical and physiological growth and by native tendencies. Training and conditioning are subsidiary to these two fundamental elements.

CHAPTER XII

CONCLUSION

Comparison with Former Studies

Biographical studies. — As yet nothing has been said with regard to former work on locomotor development. Since the methods of this study closely approximate those of biographical reports, the results are most comparable to the things recounted in the biographies. Most biographers give a brief account of the baby's motor progress, a description of his early methods of locomotion, and the ages at which he sat alone, crept, and walked. Striking indeed is the correspondence between the biographical reports of babies and the results of this study in the acquisition of motor skill. Not only do the ages at which the babies in the biographies sit, creep, stand, and walk fall well within the corresponding age ranges of this group, but the agreement in sequence of development and in accompanying motor play is almost perfect. Practically all of the peculiar modes of locomotion reported in other studies were duplicated by some baby of this group. From Preyer to Fenton the improved methods of infant care have had almost no influence on the order in which the baby develops motor skills and only slight influence on the age at which he does them.

Excellent accounts of motor development are to be found in the works of Shinn (28), Fenton (11), and Myers (24). In progress toward creeping and walking long-skirted Baby Shinn of the nineties traveled the same route at the same speed as did berompered young

Fenton of 1922, and as did the sun-suit clad babies of 1928. This is an interesting comment since Miss Shinn attributed the little girl's early awkwardness to her encumbering petticoats. Preyer (25) also stressed the hampering effect of mid-Victorian styles in baby clothes. The activities of three babies of biographies are tabulated along with the corresponding stages for babies of this group in Table VII. To avoid confusion in terminology the description of the activity as given by each biographer is included.

It will be noted that Babies Shinn and Fenton exhibited every stage of creeping that was noted by observers in this study and also that the sequence of stages was the same for these babies as for the group. Baby Myers and Baby Fenton approximately agree with the median of this group in the age at which each stage developed. Baby Shinn was considerably accelerated beyond the median and resembles Martin and Carol, who were outstanding in motor development in the present study.

Another striking resemblance is the similarity of motor play. Although pulling to a standing position by means of furniture was set as a test item in this study, it nevertheless occurred spontaneously in all of the babies. Major (22), Shinn, Myers, and Fenton all describe it as a play response in their babies, and both Shinn and Fenton report play with the toes. Mrs. Fenton writes that up until 28 weeks her baby paid no attention to his toes, although she often tried to get him interested in them. But one day "he caught sight of his foot, made a dive for it, and pulled it to his mouth. . . . From this time on his toes were among his most fascinating playthings." The suddenness of motor development was noted by both Preyer and Shinn. The former re-

TABLE VII

Comparison of Present Study and Biographical Studies

Baby Shinn		Baby Myers		Baby Fenton		Median of Babies in Present Study	
Activity	Age in Weeks	Activity	Age in Weeks	Activity	Age in Weeks	Activity	Age in Weeks
Sit propped on lounge	16	Sit on lap	16	Sit propped with pillow	14	Sit on lap	18.5
Roll	26+	Roll off blanket	25			Roll	29
Sprawl and wriggle	19	Pivot on shoulders	25	Make vigorous crawling movements	21	Swim	25
Sit alone on floor	26	Sit alone	30	Sit alone in carriage	17	Sit alone on floor 1 minute	31
Get on hands and knees	32	Get on hands and toes	32			"Suspension bridge" (8 babies)	38.5

Draw forward on stomach to reach toy; half sprawl, half creep	33			Crawl 1 foot for toy	31	Rock or pivot on stomach; some progress	35
Creep backward by pushing with hands	35	Creep backward	41	Creep; as likely to go backward as forward	42	Scoot backward pushing with hands	39.5
Real creeping	36	Creep forward well	42	Scuttle ahead rapidly	43	Creep	44.5
Pull to stand	38	Pull to stand in carriage	44	Pull to stand in play pen	39	Pull to stand	45
Lower self carefully from standing position	41	Sit down easily when standing by person	46			Sit from stand	47
Stand alone	45	Stand and squat	53			Stand alone	62
Walk alone	50	Walk 15 feet	54	Walk across room	56	Walk alone	64

ported that his son had taken only a few steps until his 66th week when he ran around a large table, staggering but not falling. Mrs. Fenton writes, "Now in his 56th week, came sudden security. We were visiting in an unfamiliar house, full of objects most alluring to baby eyes. The baby stood beside me, gazing with interest at the high lights on a curiously carved chair that stood on the farther side of the large room, and suddenly, almost before I realized what was happening, he had walked unwaveringly across the room and was fingering the interesting knobs and corners happily." Both Preyer and Fenton stress the instinctive character of walking.

Experimental studies. — Of experimental studies there have been relatively few. In 1881 Vierordt (37) devised a clever, ink-writing overshoe whereby he studied the length, width, and angle of step in two children at the ages of 2½ and 4½ years, and in one adult. On the three cases he found a lengthening of step, a narrowing in relative width, and an increase in angle of step with age. The first two findings are in keeping with those of the present walking study. The tendency of the adult of 1880 to out-toe more than the child may have been due to Victorian prejudices against pigeon-toeing or to the style of shoe worn fifty years ago.

More recently Jones (17) set out to study the development of head support and sitting alone together with other "behavior patterns." The former she gave up entirely because she was unable to score the baby in regard to head support. The criterion that she used in the sitting test was that the baby sit unsupported for five seconds. The age at which 50 per cent of the babies were able to pass this test was 225 days or 32 weeks. This age is one week older than the median age at which babies of this group sat unsupported for sixty seconds.

In her study of locomotion in infants Burnside (8) discovered three main stages in locomotion: crawling on the abdomen, creeping, and walking alone. Her report contains fine camera-lucida drawings that show the different stages of progress very clearly. Her cases, however, were so few and her ages so scattered that she missed several interesting and important stages of locomotor development.

In his study of high school and college men Dougan (10) found angles of gait of 6.1 degrees and 7.2 degrees. He noted that angles were greater when the subjects were fatigued from football practice, and he believed that angles increased with age as balancing became more difficult. The decrease of angle in babyhood and early childhood is an interesting adjunct to his findings.

Observation and relational studies of locomotion.— Trettein (31) in 1900 gave a very clear and extensive description of postures and of the manner of crawling hitching, creeping, and climbing in the newborn baby. His material was obtained from detailed questionnaires that were sent to parents.

Bauer (6) calls attention to a creeping phenomenon in the newborn infant. When the baby is placed on his stomach on a table he usually kicks and waves. If he is given something to kick against, a board or the examiner's hands, his vigorous kicking sends him forward a few inches. Fenton has noted this early creeping, and it was observed in several babies in this study, notably on Virginia Ruth who kicked the examiner's abdomen hard enough to shove away the table on which she was lying. Like sucking, Bauer considers this reaction a complex instinctive act, the adequate stimulus for which is pressure on the soles of the feet.

Variot has recently made extensive studies of locomotion in infants. From reports of prelocomotion in eighty babies he found that only thirty-eight progressed in some way before they walked alone. Of these, seventeen crept on hands and knees, thirteen hitched along in the sitting posture, and three trotted on all fours. More than half of the babies walked without any preliminary creeping stage. No case of this sort was found in the present study.

Variot and Gotcu (34, 35) obtained records of the ages at walking of five hundred French children. The results can be easily summarized in tabular form:

		Per Cent of 500 Cases
Variation in age at walking	11–14 mo.	67.00
Variation in height at walking	71–76 cm.	68.50
Variation in weight at walking	9.0–9.6 kg.	67.00
Variation in number of teeth	4–8	67.15

Nutrition	Age of Walking Alone in Months	Per Cent of 500 Cases
Breast feeding only	11–14	82.00
Breast and bottle mixed	11–14	68.58
Bottle only	11–14	61.45

They also report that girls walk somewhat earlier than boys. Babies with birth weight under 3,000 grams and those with weight over 3,750 grams walked somewhat later than babies who weighed 3,000 to 3,750 grams at birth. Probably the reason is that the unusually small babies are premature, and perhaps large babies are more subject to birth injury.

Variot concludes that although there is a large hereditary factor in walking (cf. the discussion of the talent hypothesis), nutrition, weight, and height are of little importance. He considers age the primary factor, but not age in itself so much as age in the sense of maturation. He advances a physiological notion that the development of the nervous system and particularly that of the centers for coordination in locomotion are the indispensable conditions for walking, a skill that develops independently of height and subordinate to age. He also attributes the creeping of the prelocomotor phase to the fact that development of the lower limbs lags behind that of the trunk. His view has a counterpart in the hypothesis of maturation set forth in the present paper.

Studies of the relation of walking age to intelligence and school success have been cited in Chapter IX. In the studies of Terman (29), Abt (1), and Aoki (3) age of walking was determined by the mother's report. The correlations are in general positive and low, that obtained by Aoki, +.53, being highest. No other author has reported a correlation between school grades and age of walking, but since the relation of walking age to intelligence as found by Abt, Adler, and Bartelme is considerably lower, one wonders if there may not be factors in the Japanese school curriculum or other chance factors operating to make the correlation spuriously high. The wider range of cases made available through the records of the Institute of Juvenile Research is sufficient to account for the fact that their correlations are higher than those found in this study.

Techniques for studying locomotion. — Several interesting variations of Vierordt's method of recording footprints have been devised. Burnside's use of an inked pad has already been mentioned. Dougan (10) used special hobnailed shoes to obtain the imprint of his subjects' feet. Wolff (39) has used a powder technique similar to that employed in this study to obtain her data on the development of the foot as an organ of locomotion. The method allows her to study the development of impulse points, i.e., points that receive the greatest portion of the weight in walking. The earliest impulse point to appear is the print of the heel; prints of the ball, the mid-foot, and the big toe, respectively, appear later.

A totally different technique has been devised by Schwartz and Voeth (26) for studying gaits in the adult. A small kymographic spool and needle are enclosed in a little box that is strapped to the small of the back. The movement of each limb displaces the lever-like needle, and the gait is represented by a continuous line. Limping and other abnormalities of gait show very clearly in the tracings.

Mechanism of walking. — At intervals throughout the German literature there appear articles on the mechanisms of walking, with drawings showing the position of each foot at each moment of the step and curves of the arcs through which the hips and legs swing. Such material is to be found in Hermann's *Handbuch der Physiologie* (15), and in the works of Jendrassik (16) Bois Reymond (7), and Kraus (18). Hermann also reports step length for adults as varying between .85 and .39 meters and walking speed between 2.39 and .38 meters per second.

Relevant material on locomotion from the animal field. — From the literature of comparative neurology and animal behavior come many studies that lend support to the maturation theory set forth in this work. From his extensive work on amblystoma Coghill (9) casts doubt on the commonly accepted theory that behavior patterns are built up from a linking of reflexes. To the contrary he finds that behavior springs forth fully formed or integrated and breaks up into reflexes later. He states that locomotion has a specific neural counterpart and holds that the locomotor pattern forms according to laws of growth within the nervous sytem. The neural pattern is primary, the behavior, secondary.

To be sure, the human infant is a more complex organism than amblystoma punctatum, possessed of a large repertoire of acts at birth, the earliest age at which he can be observed. Individuation of some reflexes has already occurred. Nevertheless, the sudden appearance of integrated locomotor skills that the babies apparently had never practiced is in accordance with the development of locomotion in amblystoma. The law of integration first and individuation into reflexes later probably applies to babies as well as to lower vertebrates. Certainly it is impossible, even by prolonged and careful observation, to see the building up of locomotion from reflexes. Coghill's interpretation is in perfect agreement with these observations.

The importance of maturation of the nervous system for behavior has been pointed out by Addison (2), who says: "The development of motor activities of the young rat is closely correlated with that of the cerebellum, and the animal is in full possession of its motor powers when the cerebellum has attained its mature arrangement."

From Avery's (5) catalogue of responses of fetal guinea pigs it appears that the same general order and sequence of motor development holds for animals and humans alike. The earliest motor responses of the guinea pig were kicking and grasping, which were manifested by 50-day-old fetuses. Ten days later rolling and crawling had developed, and the 63-day-old pigs were able to stand and walk. At this time the front legs were stronger than the hind legs.

Guinea pigs develop at a much more rapid rate than babies, and hence the transition from stage to stage was a matter of hours or minutes with them, whereas in the baby it required days and weeks. All the stages observed in the guinea pig occurred similarly in the baby, and the weakness of the guinea pig's hind parts is comparable with the anterior-posterior trend of motor development in the baby. A comparison of the two studies brings the suggestion not only that a pattern of motor development obtains within a species but that it holds for the whole animal scale.

Tilney and Casamajor (30) studied behavior and myelinogeny simultaneously in newborn kittens. They found a definite order of sequence in behavior development and ascribed it to the myelinization of the nervous system. Their work favors the maturation hypothesis.

Finally, the works of Lui and Laughton give some clue as to the nervous mechanism regulating locomotion. In experiments on cats and dogs Laughton (20) found that the caudal two-thirds of the thalamus had to be intact for locomotion to take place normally. Lui (21) studied the cerebellum of the infant and the dog progressively until walking was manifested. He also studied the ewe and the pigeon, both of which walk at birth. He found progressive changes in the cerebellar arrangements that consisted largely of a disappearance of the external granular layer, a marked increase in the molecular layer, and an increase in the protoplasm of Purkinje cells whereby they progress from a pyramidal to a globular form, the nucleus migrating from the lower part of the cell toward the center. These changes have taken place in the infant by 18 months, which is about the age of walking alone. Similar changes take place in the dog, whereas the lamb is born with a more highly developed cerebellum. Lui concludes that not only does the age of walking coincide with cerebellar development but also that differences in development at birth make for differences in locomotor skill of the newborn of different species.

The maturation hypothesis set fourth in this monograph is, therefore, in perfect accord with the results of biologists and neurologists obtained on both animals and humans.

CONCLUSIONS

PATTERN OF MOTOR DEVELOPMENT

1. Motor development, quite apart from age, follows a pattern that has five major orders. They may be described more or less adequately as: (a) development of passive postural control; (b) development of active postural control; (c) active efforts toward locomotion; (d) locomotion by creeping and walking with support; (e) walking alone.

2. Each major order of development has several stages. There is some shifting in sequence of stages within an order, but there is no transposition of a stage from one order to another.

3. The motor play of a baby at any age is in accordance with the activities of the order of development in which he is at the time.

4. The pattern-like character of motor development seems best accounted for on the basis of maturation because there are anatomical and physiological correlates with motor development, and because the sudden appearance of new stages points toward the maturation hypothesis.

INDIVIDUALITY IN MOTOR DEVELOPMENT

1. There is great variability among the babies in the

age at which each passes through the different stages of motor development.

2. There are great differences among the babies in their delight in motor play and in the amount and strenousness of their activity.

3. Individual differences in motor development among babies can best be accounted for on the basis of a motor "talent" or predisposition toward good coordination for the following reasons: (a) Motor differences appear at birth or shortly thereafter and persist throughout the first two years. (b) Differences in spontaneous practice of the babies can be accounted for only on the basis of differences in their delight in motor activity, conditioning, or parental training. (c) It is inconceivable that parents would train babies in the types of motor play in which they indulge, even if they did train them for creeping or walking.

SPECIFIC PHASES OF MOTOR DEVELOPMENT

1. Progress toward creeping goes through the following stages: (a) lifting the head, chin free, when on the stomach; (b) lifting the head, chest free, when on the stomach; (c) knee pushing or swimming; (d) rolling; (e) rocking, pivoting, worming along; some method of making progress; (f) scooting backward by using the hands; (g) creeping forward.

2. Progress toward assuming an upright posture goes through the following stages: (a) lifting the head when lying on the back; (b) sitting alone momentarily; (c) sitting alone; (d) standing holding to furniture; (e) pulling self to standing position by means of furniture; (f) sitting from the standing posture.

3. Progress toward walking goes through the following stages: (a) an early period of stepping; (b) stand-

ing with the support of a person; (c) walking with help, led by a person; (d) standing alone; (e) walking alone.

4. When the child walks alone he shows increase in skill in the following ways: (a) gradual increase in walking speed; (b) increase in length of step; (c) decrease in width of step; (d) decrease in angle of step; (e) increasing tendency toward straight rather than out-toeing steps.

APPENDIXES

APPENDIX 1

Facsimile of the Anthropometric Measurements Record Sheet

INSTITUTE OF CHILD WELFARE | **INFANT STUDY** | **UNIVERSITY OF MINNESOTA**

ANTHROPOMETRIC MEASUREMENTS

Name ____________

Date ____________

Hour ____________

Birthdate ____________

Age in weeks ____________

		CRYING			EYE MOVT.			ARM MOVT			LEG MOVT.			DIGESTIVE	MOUTH MOVT.		VOCALIZATION		BODY AND HEAD MOVT.
		Screaming	Fussing		Random looking	Watching		Random waving	Withdrawal, w ; push, p.		Random kicking	Defence kick ; def. flex		Belch, b ; hiccough, h ; gas, g ; vomit, v ; regurgitate, r ; defecation, d ; urination, u.	Sucking		Sneeze, s. ; cough, c.		
Fronto-occipital cir.																			
Supraorbito-occ. cir.																			
Neck cir.																			
Fronto-occipital diam.																			
Supraorbito-occ. diam.																			
Mento-occipital																			
Orbito-auricular																			
Ear																			
Nasion-menton																			
Biparietal																			
Bimalar																			
Bigonial																			
Bicondylar																			
Undress																			
Bideltoid																			
Nipple																			
Xiphisternal																			
Tenth rib																			
Umbilical																			
Iliacal																			
Biceps																			
Maximum forearm																			
Minimum forearm																			
Wrist																			
Hand																			

APPENDIX 2

Facsimile of Mothers' Daily Record Sheet, Form II, Used between 13 and 32 Weeks

13

INSTITUTE OF CHILD WELFARE **INFANT STUDY—DAILY RECORD SHEET, FORM II.** **UNIVERSITY OF MINNESOTA**

Child's name Date Birth date Age weeks and days. Weight Room temperature

Feeding Record

Number of feedings in 24 hours

Average length of each nursing period

At which feeding did baby fail to take usual amount?

Which feeding did baby refuse?

Note any irregularity in nursing

Additional foods:

Kind	Hour of Feeding	Amount Taken	Like Indicated by	Dislike Indicated by

As new foods are offered state briefly how you prepare them

Personal Habits

Number of stools in 24 hours

Stool character. ☐ soft; ☐ formed; ☐ watery; ☐ curds

Stool color. ☐yellow ☐ brown; ☐ green ☐ used pot

Night sleep From ____ to ____; from ____ to ____

Day naps From ____ to ____; from ____ to ____; from ____ to ____

Crying Spells	From— to—	From— to—	From— to—	From— to—
Intensity of Crying Apparent Cause	Fuss cry scream	Fuss cry scream	Fuss cry scream	Fuss cry scream
Attempted Reliefs (Underline those tried and encircle s or f too indicate succeeded or failed in quieting baby.)	Feeding s f Changing s f Took baby up s f Ignored baby s f	Feeding s f Changing s f Took baby up s f Ignored baby s f	Changing s f Feeding s f Took baby up s f Ignored baby s f	Feeding s f Changing s f Took baby up s f Ignored baby s f
Other Reliefs	s f	s f	s f	s f
Other Reliefs	s f	s f	s f	s f

Signs of Development. Check. Add Notes

☐ Turned from side to back or stomach
☐ Turned from stomach to back or back to stomach
☐ Rolled from back to back or stomach to stomach
☐ Sits when propped with pillows
☐ Pushes self to sitting posture in crib
☐ Sits alone. How long?
☐ Pusheswith toes when lying on stomach
☐ Creeps or hitches
☐ Pushes feet against lap when held erect, feet touching
☐ Stepping movements when held with feet touching table
☐ Pulls self to standing posture in crib
☐ Stands holding to furniture

☐ Walks holding to furniture
☐ Stands alone ☐ Walks alone
☐ Looks for fallen object
☐ Throws objects to floor ☐ Throws object for noise
☐ Reacts to self in mirror
☐ Laughs out loud
Recognized ☐ mother; ☐ father; ☐ friend, ☐ stranger
Quieted by ☐ voice; ☐ caress; ☐ picking up
Music: ☐ listens; ☐ stops cry; ☐ coos; ☐ bounces up and down
☐ Waves bye-bye ☐ Plays peek-a-boo.
☐ Plays pat-a-cake

☐ Handles spoon for eating
☐ Holds cup for drinking
☐ Leafs through magazines
Describe other tricks of the baby and other things done in apparent imitation of adult activity

Sucks thumb: ☐ Constantly; ☐ frequently; ☐ occasionally
☐ Holds bottle ☐ Grasps object
☐ Reaches for object
☐ Puts object in mouth
☐ Plays with object
☐ Plays with own hands
☐ Plays with own toes
☐ Kicks in bath ☐ Splash in bath ☐ Cried in bath
☐ Holds out arms to come
☐ Responds to own name

☐ Knows brother's or sisters name
☐ Knows objects by name
☐ Responds to words not accompanied by gestures
List words child used with meaning; Dada occurs as a natural sound, but is a word only when used to mean the father

How does baby react when adults come near his crib?

How does baby react when a child comes near his crib?

Favorite toy

General Conduct for entire day: ☐Very cross; ☐ somewhat fretful; ☐ quiet and docile, ☐ somewhat playful, ☐ very playful and active.

General physical state: ☐ Rash, ☐ head sweat; ☐ nose runs; ☐ drooling; ☐ appearance of new tooth.

Note. If fright or temper tantrums occur during the day fill in the back of this sheet. Note other unusual occurrences.

APPENDIX 3

Items on Mothers' Daily Record Sheet, Form I, Used between 3 and 12 Weeks*

Signs of Development

Underline or check any of the items below which occurred once or more during the day.

Mark those occurring during the bath with a B. Add notes if you desire.

__ Coughed; __ sneezed; __ stretched; __ tears

Turned from side to back or stomach

Turned from back to stomach or stomach to back

Rolled completely from back to back or stomach to stomach

Lifted head when on stomach; chin up

Lifted head when on stomach; chest up

Tensed muscles to be lifted

Listened: __ to voice; __ to music

Babbled: __ when talked to; __ when no one was around

Gestures: __ of negation; __ withdrawal; __ pain

Smiled: __ from bodily contentment; __ when smiled at

Laughed out loud

Reactions to being dressed and undressed (describe)

Bath: __ liked; __ disliked; __ splashed; __ cried

__ Blinked at sound; __ startled by sound; __ cried at sound

Noticed: __ light; __ object; __ person

Recognized: __ mother; __ father; __ friends; __ strangers

Puts object in mouth

Makes defensive hand movements

Sucked: __ hand; __ thumb; __ clothing

Reached for object

Grasped object not put against palm

Averts head from strong light

Played: __ with hands; __ with toes

Quieted: __ by voice; __ by caress; __ by picking up

Note other signs of development

General conduct for entire day: (check most descriptive phrase) __ very cross; __ somewhat fretful; __ quiet and docile; __ cheerful, somewhat playful; __ very active and playful

General physical state: (check anything you noticed) belched: __ fussy, __ not fussy; passed gas: __ fussy, __ not fussy; __ had rash; __ head sweat; __ nose run; teething: __ irritable, __ drooling

* Form I was similar to Form II, on the opposite page. There was space for a complete record of feeding and habits of sleep and elimination.

APPENDIX 4

ITEMS ON MOTHERS' DAILY RECORD SHEET, FORM III, USED BETWEEN 32 AND 52 WEEKS*

Regular Daily Schedule

Night sleep from ______ to ______; from ______ to ______
__ Usually sleeps soundly; __ usually wakeful
Day naps from ______ to ______; from ______ to ______;
from ______ to ______
__ Usually sleeps soundly; __ usually wakeful
Hours of bath ______ __ sponge; __ tub
Usual number of stools per day ______
Stools: __ usually formed; __ usually soft
Approximate no. of hours per day spent outdoors ______
Approximate no. of hours per day left to amuse self ______
Approximate no. of hours per day spent with children ______
Approximate no. of hours per day spent with adults ______
Approximate no. of hours per day spent in baby swing ______
Approximate no. of hours per day spent on floor and allowed the range of the room or of the house ______
Approximate no. of waking hours per day kept in crib ______
Approximate no. of hours per day kept in pen ______
__ Day naps out of doors
__ Taken out in carriage for walk daily
__ Plays in pen out of doors

Self Help in Eating. Check. Add Notes

__ Takes bottle in and out of mouth
__ Holds bottle entirely for eating
__ Reaches toward dish of food
__ Feeds self cereal or vegetable by dipping up handfuls
__ Feeds self with spoon
__ Helps to hold cup for drinking
__ Holds cup alone for drinking, using both hands
__ Holds cup alone for drinking, using one hand
__ Fusses for food upon seeing others eat

PECULIARITIES IN EATING

__ Spits food out of mouth
__ Crams mouth too full of food to swallow
__ Takes very small bites; minces
__ Holds food in mouth without swallowing
Add notes on help or peculiarities ______

* This form provided for a record of the regular daily food schedule, daily departures from the usual schedule, and a daily rating of the baby's general behavior.

Self Help in Personal Habits

Bowel control (encircle)	none;	partial;	complete
Bladder control (encircle)	none;	partial;	complete

Bath

__ Splashes in bath
__ Rubs soap on body
__ Rubs body with washcloth or towel
__ Turns on water in tub
__ Pulls out plug to let water drain out
Others ______

Dressing and Undressing

__ Helps to pull stockings off
__ Pulls arms out of sleeves without help
__ Pulls off shoes or booties
__ Pulls off hat or cap
__ Thrusts arms into sleeves without help
__ Tries to pull stockings on
__ Tries to put shoes on
__ Tries to pull dress or sweater over head
__ Places hat or cap on head

Cleanliness

__ Makes sign when wet or soiled
__ Examines hands when wet or sticky
__ Wipes hands when dirty or sticky

Gross Motor Control

__ Rolls back to stomach or from stomach to back
__ Rolls completely two or three times in succession
__ Creeps or hitches
__ Crawls; goes on all fours
__ Pulls self to sitting posture
__ Pulls self to standing posture
__ Stands holding to furniture
__ Walks holding to furniture
__ Stands alone. How long? ______
__ Walks, pushing furniture in front
__ Walks alone. How many steps? ______
__ Climbs upstairs (all fours)
__ Climbs downstairs
__ Climbs on stools or chairs
__ Climbs off stools or chairs

__ Propels kiddy-car
__ Rocks in rocking chair
__ Bounces in baby swing
__ Bounces on stuffed chairs
__ Bounces or dances to music

List and describe other activities and stunts of the baby that may be classified under this heading ______________________

Describe method of creeping or crawling ______________________

Fine Motor Control

__ Picks up small objects (pins, pills, beads, etc.)
__ Pulls cork out of bottle
__ Pulls lid off of can
__ Unscrews lid of jar or can
__ Piles up blocks (encircle number) 2 3 4 5 6
__ Turns pages of magazine
__ Marks with pencil
__ Pushes button to turn on light
__ Puts lid on box
__ Drops beads into bottle
__ Puts lid on can
__ Puts cork in bottle
__ Blows horn or whistle

Other reactions that might be classified under this head ______________________

Favorite Toys. List

____

Comprehension of Language

__ Turns when own name is called
__ Knows brother's or sister's name (looks for them)
__ Knows object by name (points or looks at it)
__ Obeys simple command, "Put it down"
__ Points to light at command
__ Takes object out of mouth at command
__ Waves bye-bye at command
__ Plays peeka-boo at command
__ Points to eyes, nose, mouth at command
__ Plays pat-a-cake at command
__ Kisses at command
__ Shakes hands at command

List words that child apparently comprehends and explain briefly the situation that leads you to think he understood ____________

Use of Speech

Inflection

__ Coos or babbles in contented tones
__ Gurgles or chuckles in tones of delight or pleasure
__ Jabbers or babbles in scolding tones
__ Yells or squeals in excited tones (not crying)
__ Yells or cries as if angry
__ Utters plaintive cry as if disappointed or displeased
__ Calls or yells (not cry) apparently to draw attention of others
Others ____________

____

Imitation of Sounds

__ Repeats ba-ba or equivalent syllable after parent
__ Repeats word after parent. List words ____________

____

Other imitative sounds ____________

____

Spontaneous Talking

__ Jabbers or babbles to doll or other object
__ Jabbers or babbles to other persons
__ Invents word or syllable to mean a certain object, "da-ta" to mean "lady"
List ____________

____

Use of Language for Needs

__ Uses noise, sound, or word as sign for bowel movement
__ Uses word or sound to ask for drink
__ Uses word or sound to ask for food
List others ____________

____

Conversation with Meaning

__ Says childish words (as bow-wow; moo-moo, etc.) appropriately. List words ____________

____

____

__ Uses adult words appropriately (as milk, doll, etc.)
List words ____________

____

Development of Senses

Vision

__ Notices objects out of window
__ Notices birds
__ Notices insects (bees, flies, ants, etc.)
__ Notices small objects (bead, pin, pill, etc.)
__ Notices a beam of sunlight
__ Notices shadows
__ Looks at pictures with interest
__ Apparently identifies a picture as an object
__ Reacts to mirror image (describe) ____________________
____
__ Looks at distant objects (trees, etc.)
__ Recognizes father or mother at a distance (across the street)

Taste

Reaction to sweet ____________________
Reaction to sour ____________________
Reaction to bitter ____________________
Reaction to salt ____________________

Smell

__ Puts flower to nose and sniffs
__ Reaction to bad odor (describe) ____________________
____

Touch

Reaction to fur ____________________
Reaction to velvet ____________________
Reaction to sand ____________________
Reaction to stickiness ____________________
Reaction to tickle ____________________

Heat and Cold

Reaction to cold food in mouth ____________________
Reaction to cold water on body ____________________
Reaction to very warm object (hot dish or metal not hot enough to burn)
____

Sense of Balance

Reaction to riding on street car ____________________
Reaction to riding in automobile ____________________
____

Reaction to riding in perambulator ____________________
Reaction to sliding on incline ____________________
Reaction to being bounced on knee ____________________
Reaction to being tossed in air ____________________

SOUND

Reaction to crash or bang ____________________
Reaction to music ____________________
Reaction to watch tick ____________________
__ Recognizes persons by sounds, as mother's voice
__ Recognizes objects by sounds, as sound of his food being prepared

Other Play Reactions

__ Puts fingers into adult's eyes, nose, mouth, etc.
__ Tries to pry adult's closed eyes open
__ Pulls spectacles off adult's face
__ Ceases to pull spectacles off adult's face
__ Hunts for objects put out of sight
__ Throws objects to floor, looks after them
__ Pulls hat or paper off head
__ Recognizes signs of going "bye-bye"
Other play activities ____________________

Personality Reactions

__ Is timid or afraid of strangers
__ Ceases to be timid with strangers
__ Is friendly with strangers (goes to them)
__ Expresses disappointment if others go out without taking him
Describe signs of affection ____________________

Name objects feared ____________________

Describe reactions to adults ____________________

Describe reactions to children ____________________

APPENDIX 5

Last Page of All Three Forms of Mothers' Daily Record Sheet

	Time	Cause	Behavior	Behavior of Persons Caring for Baby
Possible frights	Hour ______	What was baby doing ______	Screaming ______	Snatched child from danger
	Place ______	______	Catches breath ______	______
	Baby under whose care	______	Rigidity ______	Screamed ______
	______	Describe situation producing fright ______	Time required to calm baby ______	Was frightened and nervous
	Was baby in danger ______			______
	Was baby injured ______	______	______	Was calm ______
				Behavior of other persons present ______
Anger	**Time**	**Cause**	**Behavior**	How was baby quieted ______
	Hour ______	What was baby doing ______	Screaming ______	______
	Place ______	______	Kicking ______	______
	Baby under whose care	______	Throwing arms about ______	______
	______	Describe anger producing situation ______	______	How long did outburst last
	______		______	______
Accidents	**Time**	How did accident happen	How serious was accident	How long did it require to quiet baby ______
	Hour ______	______	______	
	Place ______	Describe ______	______	How long for complete recovery from wound ______
	Baby under whose care	______	______	
	______	______	______	______

Signs of affection

Patted mother's breast ____________ Other signs of affection ____________

Patted mother's face ____________

Whimpered at strange face ____________

Held out arms to come to mother ____________

Habits and Training

Bowel control: Describe methods used to teach child bowel control. What progress have you made? ____________

Thumb sucking: Describe degree and frequency of thumb or finger sucking, and state whether an attempt has been made to break habit, describe methods, and state progress ____________

Other training attempted ____________

Upsets in family schedule ____________

APPENDIX 6

Dramatis Personae

Baby	No. of Siblings	Father: Occupation	Father: Education	Father: Descent	Father: Talent or Hobby	Mother: Premarital Occupation	Mother: Education	Mother: Descent	Mother: Talent or Hobby
Nathaniel	1 m	University professor	Ph.D.	English	No information	No information	B.A.	English	Writing
Matthew	1 f	Sales engineer	B.S.	English	Military training	Manager of employment bureau	Some college training	English	No information
Donovan	1 m	Clerk	Some high school training	Scotch-Irish	Dancing	Telephone operator	Some high school training	German	Sketching and drawing
Doris	1 m	Inspector of long distance telephone lines	Some high school training	English	Study and sports	Supervisor of telephone operators	Some high school training	German	Sketching and drawing
Sibyl	2 f	Civil engineer	B.S.	English	No information	No information	B.A.	English	No information
Virginia Ruth	2 f	University professor	Ph.D.	English	No information	Interior decorator	B.S.	English	No information
Thorwald (Torey)	0	Insurance salesman	Some college training	English	No information	Teacher	B.A.	Scandinavian	No information
James D.	1 m	Radio broker	High school graduate	English-Irish	Electrical engineering	In newspaper advertising	Some college training	Irish-French	Dramatics
David	1 m	Attorney	LL.B.	English	No information	No information	High school; business college	Scandinavian	No information
Margaret	1 f 1 m	Minister	B.A.; B.D.	Dutch-German	Athletics	No information	B.A.	English	Music and painting
Waldemar (Walley)	1 f	Traveling salesman	No information	No information	Athletics	No information	No information	Scandinavian	No information
Judy	1 f	Dental technician	Some high school training	Scotch-Irish	No information	Stenographer and bookkeeper	High school graduate	Scandinavian	No information

Irene May	0	Manager of bus lines	No information	No information	No information	No information	No information	No information	No information
Maurice	2 f 1 m	Memorial craftsman and marble dealer	College training in Russia	Russian-Hebrew	Art and sculpture	In medical social service	Some college training	Russian-Hebrew	Business
Edith Ann	1 m 1 f	University professor	Ph.D.	English	No information	Teacher	M.A.	English, French, Dutch	No information
Carol	1 f 1 m	Lumber salesman	Some college training	German	Sports	Bank teller	B.A.; music conservatory	English	Music
Rexroad }	1 f	Merchant	No information	Hebrew	No information	No information	No information	Hebrew	No information
Maxfield } (cousins)	0	Merchant	No information	Hebrew	No information	No information	No information	Hebrew	No information
Fred } Winifred } (twins)	1 f 2 m	University professor	Ph.D.	Scandinavian	Sports	Teacher and secretary	Some college training	English	Writing
Martin	1 f 1 m	Furniture manufacturer	High school graduate	German	Gardening	No information	High school graduate	No information	No information
Quentin	1 m	Machinist	Some high school; technical school	German	No information	In clerical work; music teacher	High school graduate; music	German	Music
Peter } Patricia } (twins)	1 f	Traveling salesman	Some college training	Swiss	Golf	Stenographer	High school graduate; business college	English-French	No information
Harvey	1 m	Merchant	Some college training	English	No information	No information	B.A.	English	Aesthetic dancing
Lawrence (Larry)	1 f 1 m	Physician	M.D.	English	Noinformation	In chatauqua work	Some college training	English	Singing and music

APPENDIX 7

First Order Skills (Age of Development in Weeks)

	Chin Up When on Stomach	Chest Up When on Stomach	Stepping	Adjust for Lifting	Knees Straight	Sit on Lap
Martin	3	18	14	..	13	19
Carol	3	9	..	19	10	15
Max	3	9	11	14	15	14
Virginia Ruth	2	3	..	15	19	19
Sibyl	1	5	11	22	16	20
David	5	7	18	18	19	18
James D.	2	5	19	18	..	19
Harvey	7	10	11	14	15	13
Winifred	10	19	15	15	19	19
Quentin	7	10	8	14	14	18
Maurice	3	9	13	21	13	14
Judy	2	3	18	18	18	18
Irene May	9	10	13	18	..	21
Peter	2	10	15	14	23	21
Walley	5	9	15	18	..	15
Fred	10	18	15	14	15	18
Donovan	2	5	12	..	14	21
Patricia	10	7	11	14	14	23
Torey	2	2	..	14	21	18
Larry	10	11	10	13	..	19
Doris	1	5	6	..	10	13
Edith Ann	3	14	13	14	23	23
Median	3	9	13	15	15	18.5
Range of middle 50 per cent	2–7	5–10	11–15	14–18	13–19	15–19.5

APPENDIX 7—*Continued*

SECOND AND THIRD ORDER SKILLS (AGE OF DEVELOPMENT IN WEEKS)

	Sit Alone Momentarily	Knee Push or Swim	Rolling	Stand Well with Help	Sit Alone 1 Minute	Some Progress on Stomach	Scoot Backward
Martin	24	18	30	27	25	25	29
Carol	29	21	27	25	30	..	37
Max	25	23	29	29	27	27	..
Virginia Ruth	24	38	25	29	34	..	41
Sibyl	29	29	20	30	34	..	45
David	27	18	25	27	27	31	34
James D.	28	22	33	35	31	37	38
Harvey	20	25	35	29	33	41	37
Winifred	25	25	24	29	27	38	42
Quentin	27	22	29	29	33	35	38
Maurice	20	27	36	34	35	41	..
Judy	29	21	30	34	34	34	47
Irene May	25	37	26	34	33	38	46
Peter	25	25	..	31	31	..	46
Walley	20	25	27	37	34	42	41
Fred	20	27	28	32	..	42	..
Donovan	25	35	35	29	35	43	46
Patricia	25	23	25	33	29	27	34
Torey	23	29	..	31	29	35	34
Larry	25	25	32	..	25	..	..
Doris	20	35	..	21	..	37	..
Edith Ann	21	27	30	..	34	39	..
Median	25	25	29	29.5	31	37	39.5
Range of middle 50 per cent	20.5–26	22–27	25–32	29–33	27–34	32.5–41	34–45.5

APPENDIX 7—*Continued*

FOURTH AND FIFTH ORDER SKILLS (AGE OF DEVELOPMENT IN WEEKS)

	Stand Holding to Furniture	Creep	Walk When Led	Pull to Stand	Walk Holding to Furniture (Mothers' Reports)	Stand Alone	Walk Alone
Martin	35	32	29	33	35	50	50
Carol	45	41	37	45	38	49	50
Max	33	35	25	38	..	49	54
Virginia Ruth	41	41	41	49	43	54	54
Sibyl	42	45	37	..	40	58	58
David	37	35	34	37	38	54	60
James D.	45	43	45	45	46	60	60
Harvey	42	41	42	..	52	62	62
Winifred	37	45	41	42	40	62	62
Quentin	42	40	38	42	42	62	64
Maurice	42	42	45	50	46	58	66
Judy	42	49	45	49	..	58	66
Irene May	41	50	45	44	46	66	66
Peter	42	45	49	..	..	62	66
Walley	47	45	54	50	54	66	68
Fred	42	45	46	52	45	70	70
Donovan	49	50	50	47	..	62	70
Patricia	49	48	45	50	..	70	70
Torey	42	44	72	47	45	74	74
Larry	49	49	54	..	..	76	76
Doris	42	45	44	50	46	..	..
Edith Ann	46	43	..	..	52	66	66
Median	42	44.5	45	47	45	62	64
Range of middle 50 per cent	41–45	41–45	37.5–45.5	42–49.5	40–46	56–66	59–67

APPENDIX 7—*Concluded*

Motor Skills Developed by a Few Babies

	Lift Trunk by Heels and Head on Back	Rock or Surge When Sitting	Suspension Bridge When on Stomach	Lower Self from Standing
Martin	..	..	29	41
Carol	..	..	..	45
Max	..	35	34	..
Virginia Ruth	..	..	..	49
Sibyl	..	..	47	..
David	..	27	..	41
James D.	16	..	38	50
Harvey	31	..	..	46
Winifred	33	..	40	42
Quentin	28	35	39	47
Maurice	..	..	..	..
Judy	..	36	..	50
Irene May	21	32	..	..
Peter	..	45	..	45
Walley	23	33	..	47
Fred	..	35	..	..
Donovan	..	35	..	..
Patricia	19	45	..	50
Torey	..	35	..	45
Larry	..	..	..	..
Doris	..	26	..	..
Edith Ann	..	39	..	..

BIBLIOGRAPHY

BIBLIOGRAPHY

1. Abt, Adler, Bartelme. "Relationship between onset of speech and intelligence." *J. Amer. Med. Assoc.*, 93: 1354. 1929.
2. Addison, W. H. F. "The development of the Purkinje cells and of the cortical layers in the cerebellum of the albino rat." *J. Comp. Neurol.*, 21: 459–489. 1911.
3. Aoki, S. "Significance of first walking in a child's development." *Shrini Kenkyu* (Psychol. Stud.) 21, No. 1. Child Devel. Abst. Vol. I, No. 1, p. 171.
4. Atkins, Ruth E. *The measurement of intelligence in young children by an object-fitting test,* Institute of Child Welfare, University of Minnesota Monograph Series No. 5. Minneapolis: The University of Minnesota Press. 1931.
5. Avery, G. T. "Response of foetal guinea pigs prematurely delivered." *Genet. Psychol. Monog.*, 3: 245–331. 1928.
6. Bauer, J. "Das Kriechphänomen des Neugebornen." *Klin. Wochenschr.*, pp. 1468–1469. 1926.
7. Bois Reymond, R. du. "Gelenkbewegung—spezielle Mùskelphysiologie, Stehen und Gehen." *Ergeb. d. Physiol.*, 6: 244–264. 1907.
8. Burnside, Lenoire H. "Coordination in the locomotion of infants." *Genet. Psychol. Monog.*, Vol. II, No. 5, pp. 284–372. 1927.
9. Coghill, G. E. "Correlated anatomical and physiological studies of the growth of the nervous system in amphibia." *J. Comp. Neurol.*, 41: 95–152. 1926.
10. Dougan, Stanley. "The angle of gait." *Amer. J. Phys. Anthrop.*, 7: 275–279. 1924.
11. Fenton, Jessie C. *A practical psychology of babyhood.* Boston: Houghton Mifflin Co. 1925.
12. Gesell, A. *Mental growth of the preschool child.* New York: The Macmillan Co. 1926.
13. ———. "Maturation and infant behavior patterns." *Psychol. Rev.*, 36: 307–319. 1929.
14. Goodenough, Florence L. "The reliability and validity of the Wallin peg boards." *Psychol. Clin.*, 16: 199–215. 1927.
15. Hermann, L. *Handbuch der Physiologie der Bewegungsapparate*, pp. 325–344. Leipzig: Vogel. 1879.
16. Jendrassik, E. "Weitere Beiträge zur Lehre vom Gehen." *Arch. f. Physiol.*, pp. 287–322. Suppl. Bd. 1904.
17. Jones, Mary Cover. "The development of early behavior patterns in young children." *Ped. Sem. and J. Genet. Psychol.*, 33: 538–585. 1926.

18. Kraus, W. M. "Difference between muscular and neuromuscular interpretation of walking." *Arch. Neurol. and Psychiat.*, 9: 184–207. 1923.
19. Kuhlmann, F. *A handbook of mental tests.* Baltimore: Warwick & York. 1922.
20. Laughton, N. B. "Studies on nervous regulation of progression in mammals." *Amer. J. Physiol.*, 70: 358–384. 1924.
21. Lui, A. "Quelques observations sur le développment histiologique de l'écorce cérébelleuse par rapport à la faculté de se tenir debout et de marcher." *Arch. ital. biol.*, 21: 395-397. 1894.
22. Major, D. R. *First steps in mental growth.* New York: The Macmillan Co. 1906.
23. Moore, C. "The mental development of a child." *Psychol. Rev. Monog.*, No. 3. 1896.
24. Myers, Garry C. "The evolution of an infant's walking." *Ped. Sem.*, 29: 295–301. 1922.
25. Preyer, W. *The mind of the child.* New York: D. Appleton & Co. 1899.
26. Schwartz and Voeth. "Method for making graphic records of normal and pathologic gaits." *J. Amer. Med. Assoc.*, 90: 86–89. 1928.
27. Sherman and Sherman. *The Process of Human Behavior*, p. 61. New York: W. W. Norton & Co. 1929.
28. Shinn, Millicent W. *Notes on the development of a child*, Parts III and IV. Berkeley: University of California Press. 1899.
29. Terman, L. M. *et al. Genetic studies of genius*, I, 185–187. Stanford University: Stanford University Press. 1926.
30. Tilney and Casamajor. "Myelinogeny as applied to the study of behavior." *Arch. Neurol. and Psychiat.*, 12: 1–66. 1924.
31. Trettein, A. W. "Creeping and walking." *Amer. J. Psychol.*, 12: 1–57. 1900.
32. Variot, M. G. Sur les facteurs normaux et morbides qui peuvent avançer ou retarder le debut de la marche bipède chez les jeunes enfants. Bull. mém. soc. méd., 43: 353–361. 1927.
33. ———. "La prélocomotion chez le jeune enfant avant la marche bipède." *Rev. scient.*, 65: 70–74. 1927.
34. ———. Présentation de deux frères chez lesquels le debut de la marche bipède a coincidé avec une taille de 80 cent. Bull. et mém. de la soc. d'anthrop. de Paris, 8: 13–15. 1927.
35. Variot and Gotcu. Le debut de la marche bipède chez le jeune enfant, dans ses rapports avec l'âge et la taille. Bull. et mém. de la soc. d'anthrop. de Paris, 8: 17–23. 1927.
36. ———. La marche bipède le jeune enfant dans ses rapports avec le poids de naissance, le poids actuel, la dentition, l'alimentation, et le sexe. Bull. et mém. de la soc. d'anthrop. de Paris, 8: 23–30. 1927.
37. Vierordt, H. Reported by M. W. Feldman. *Antenatal and postnatal child physiology*. New York: Longmans, Green & Co. 1920.

38. Watson, John B. *Psychological Care of Infant and Child*, p. 15. New York: W. W. Norton & Co. 1928.

39. Wolff, L. X. "Development of the human foot as an organ of locomotion." *Amer. J. Dis. Child*, 37: 1212–1220. 1929.

40. Woodworth, R. S. *Psychology*. Revised edition, pp. 212–214. New York: Henry Holt & Co. 1929.

INDEX

Made in the USA
Monee, IL
26 October 2025

32968633R00144